REVISED EDITION

Emotional
Freedom

Techniques for dealing with emotional and physical distress

Garry A. Flint, Ph.D.

NeoSolTerric Enterprises
Vernon, British Columbia

National Library of Canada Cataloguing in Publication Data

Flint, Garry A., 1934-
    Emotional freedom : techniques for dealing with emotional
and physical distress

Rev. ed.
Includes bibliographical references.
ISBN 0-9685195-1-2

    1. Acupuncture points—Popular works. 2. Self-help
techniques. I. Title.

RM723.A27F54 2001   615.8'22   C2001-901174-1

Acknowledgments

This book sums up the observations and work of Gary Craig and Adrienne Fowlie (1995), who developed and successfully taught Emotional Freedom Techniques (EFT) in peak performance seminars for a number of years. This book presents these Emotional Freedom Techniques.

These methods are largely an extension of the work described by Roger Callahan (1981, 1985, 1991, 2001) and James Durlacher (1995). Callahan developed his techniques from the work of George Goodheart (1964-78). Goodheart's work is summarized by David Walther (1981, 1988). Callahan creatively and brilliantly developed this highly effective treatment that works for most mental issues. He called this therapy Callahan Techniques™, but later, changed the name to Thought Field Therapy™. Thought Field Therapy™ was praised by Charles Figley and Joyce Carbonell in their study of effective treatments of Posttraumatic Stress Disorder (Figley and Carbonell, 1996). As compared to other treatment techniques, he noted that Thought Field Therapy™ is extraordinarily powerful, can be taught to nearly anyone, appears to do no harm, does not require the clients to talk about their troubles, and is fast and long lasting (Figley, 1995). Emotional Freedom Techniques, in addition to deserving the above praises, is easier to use.

I am indebted to Gary Craig, both for his permission to summarize his work and for his support and comments. I thank my wife, Jane Flint, and my colleagues Charles Figley, Jasenn Zaejian, Marie Green, Thomas Altaffer, and Richard F. Smith for their encouragement. For global feedback, I thank Graig Burns, Shirley McGee, Fred Madryga and Lee Pulos. I extend special thanks to Dana L. Flint, Jo Willems, and Sue McCullough for their careful and detailed editing of the manuscript. In particular, I want to thank Brian Armstrong, of Really Small Vernon Press.

I give thanks to the following people for making contributions and suggestions for the second edition: Thorsten Becker, who made suggestions that simplified the method and for suggestions about the forms and format. I am thankful for David Kohn's assistance in changing the organization and editing sections of the book. I thank Robert Juran for copy-editing the final manuscript.

Contents

Foreword

I am pleased that Dr. Garry Flint has so carefully put together this useful guide to Emotional Freedom Techniques. It is a much needed resource for this exploding concept in human healing. He not only covers the basics well, but also adds his own professional innovations – something I hope many others will do as we progress upward in this healing high-rise.

Gary Craig
The Sea Ranch,
California

Introduction

This book will show you a simple five-step method that will let you heal most of your emotional issues and eliminate or control your physical pain. Naturally, there are exceptions. For the majority of people, though, the simple healing method described in this book will work.

This book shows how you can eliminate issues that get in the way of your leading a satisfying life. Using these techniques, many people can banish fear, guilt and pain from their existence. So can you.

As you will see, the technique, though detailed, basically lets you heal yourself by tapping on acupressure points. All you have to do is follow instructions. There is only one sequence of tapping points for all mental and physical issues. This eliminates the need for diagnosis and makes learning the method easy.

Hey! It's ok to have a healthy skepticism. This healing method works on skeptics, too. You don't have to understand it or even believe it. You can learn this healing method as an experiment, just to see if it works. If it works, it's a good deal. When experimenting, you should first learn the method and then start by using it with easy issues. With success, you'll become more confident that it works. It's like learning how to ride a bicycle before you ride to school. Each time you use this healing process successfully, it's like another successful experiment. Here's what you do when you do this healing method.

The basic healing method involves five steps. The first step is to identify the issue you want to become less painful. We're talking about anxiety, fear, sadness, and the like. In most cases, you'll just have to think about the issue, then, by repeating the healing method several times, you heal the issue. However, sometimes issues are more complex. When they are, you will have to look for other aspects of the complex issue. (Aspects are other similar beliefs or traumas that help cause the issue.) The chapter on identifying the aspects of complex issues can be really important if your issues are truly complex. By healing all the aspects, you heal the issue.

The second step is a procedure in which you manage memories that get in the way of the healing process. This procedure requires you to rub on a sore spot on your chest while saying an affirmation. It's the rubbing that manages the memories. The affirmation is a self-empowering statement that increases your satisfaction in life. You do this three times.

The third step in the healing process involves tapping 5 or 6 times on each point of a sequence of twelve acupressure meridian points. As you tap on each point, you remind yourself about the issue with a phrase, such as "my anxiety." You do this to keep you thinking about the issue.

When you do the fourth step, you will repeatedly tap on an acupressure point on the back of your hand. While you tap, you'll move your eyes in different ways or you'll hum and count. You do this procedure because sometimes, when it isn't done, the emotions connected to an issue do not heal. This step is called the 9-Gamut, because you run the gamut with nine interventions – eye movements, hum, count – while you are tapping on the acupressure point.

The fifth step is to repeat the third step. That's easy. But what if the technique doesn't work?

Remember that most people, including you, probably won't have to deal with this problem. You'll probably have no difficulty in healing your issues. However, if you do run into problems, you'll know fairly quickly. The emotional intensity of each issue should diminish considerably and even disappear. When that change doesn't happen, all you have to do is look at the troubleshooting chapter. There you'll see how to troubleshoot, correct, and even remove any problem or barrier getting in the way of your healing process.

Here's how the book is laid out: The first chapter gives an overview of what can be healed, followed by a chapter giving a detailed overview of the book. This chapter is really a glossary of all the concepts used in the book. Most of the concepts discussed in the glossary are treated individually in a chapter. In the next five chapters you'll learn the healing method itself. Then an experimental procedure is presented to help the reader become confident with the healing method. Next are chapters on shortcuts and troubleshooting. Then there is a summary of the healing method with an example, followed by chapters dealing with beliefs and memories, addictions, and pain. For those who like flow charts, there is a complete flow chart. For those interested, there is a chapter that teaches the healing method to your subconscious – the Innerself. If this works, then the healing process is automated and can be used by simply asking. In the appendix are lists of issues and aspects to help you and reminder aids for the healing method.

Just remember: Following the five steps in this book could rid your life of mental and physical pain and keep them away. That's a big payback for investing a little time in a small book. I think you'll find the time well spent.

Emotional *Freedom*

Chapter 1

Foiling the Wasp:
Taking the Sting Out of
What's Troubling You

Remember when, as a kid, you got stung by a wasp or a yellow jacket? The pain always went away when the stinger was pulled out. You felt a lot better. By using The Method, you can remove the sting of painful emotions from any of your Issues. In this chapter, you'll get a wide-angle view of exactly what Issues are involved in altering those painful beliefs, memories, addictions and chronic symptoms you'd rather live without.

Beliefs and memories are slightly different from addictions and chronic symptoms. Beliefs and memories are both simply memories with emotions attached to them. Addictions and chronic symptoms involve many memories and are much more complex. Change of these Issues is briefly described in this chapter. Later, there are chapters that fully describe how to use The Method to change beliefs, memories, addictions and chronic symptoms.

By using a painful belief as an example, you will obtain a general idea of how The Method is used to reduce or remove painful emotions. Changing painful memories, emotions, pictures, intrusions, nightmares, addictive urges and chronic symptoms, and so forth, are all similar to changing a painful belief. The similarity is that they are all based on a memory. You can use The Method to change the emotions connected to the memory. An example of using The Method will be given that shows how to change or remove the emotions of an unwanted belief. This will provide you with a general understanding about how The Method can be used for removing pain from other Issues.

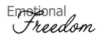

Beliefs and Memories

It is the painful emotion connected to a traumatic memory that is the part of the memory that causes problems and disrupts your life. The memory of an emotion is different from the memory of what happened. All mild and severe psychological problems, self-limiting beliefs, intrusive memories or emotions and painful traumatic memories are memories with painful memories of emotion connected to them. Again, it is painful memories of emotion connected to experiential memories that make them painful.

Let's look at beliefs as an example. It is easy to change an unwanted belief using The Method. A belief is either true or not true for you, depending upon the intensity of the positive or negative emotions attached to the belief. If a negative belief is true for you, it can pop up in your thoughts frequently. To get rid of an unwanted negative belief, you simply have to change the belief from being true to being not true. When it is not true for you, you will tend to forget about it.

Hurt, by the way, is a term that stands for all negative emotions. This will be explained further below. Unwanted beliefs are beliefs that are true for you. They are true because they have Hurt associated with them. It is the Hurt that makes the unwanted belief true. When you remove the Hurt from the belief, the belief becomes not true for you. When it is not true, it will not intrude into your thoughts. You can use The Method to remove the Hurt from a belief. You can also strengthen weak, positive beliefs, so they are totally true for you. This will be explained later.

Fears, bad feelings, thoughts and memories of bad events, including all the symptoms they cause, are memories with Hurt associated with them. So to change one of these Issues, all you have to do is use The Method to remove the Hurt from the memory. Similar to beliefs, if the painful emotions are removed from an intrusive voice, image, or "movie," they will stop occurring to you. The changed memory is not lost, and may even be more accurate or complete.

What it won't have is old Hurt associated with it. With the Hurt removed, the memory or experience will have less or no impact on your life. Without it, your life can be more satisfying.

Addictions

Addictions can be stopped. The Method eliminates addictive urges. Since all addictive urges are driven by Hurt, The Method gives you choice. You will have choice because it gives you a way to change the Hurt and neutralize your urge or craving whenever it occurs. To be sure, it takes a strong desire to make the choice to stop an addiction. It is important to do The Method before you do your addiction – before you binge eat, drink, or smoke – otherwise The Method will not work. Because of the complexity of addictions, you will be encouraged to persistently and routinely use The Method to change your addictive urges whenever they are present. The strategy for changing addictions will be described in a later chapter. Do not try to change an addictive urge while you are reading this book. First, understand how to do The Method; then build confidence that The Method will work for you by using it on less difficult Issues. Because addictive urges are sometimes more resistant to change, it is your confidence that The Method will work for you that will give you the patience and persistence necessary to change addictive urges.

Chronic Symptoms

Physical ailments, aches and pains and symptoms of chronic illnesses often have symptoms that are learned associated with them. You can use The Method to neutralize those learned and remembered painful symptoms. Also, stress causes tension in the muscles – that aggravates the Hurt caused by physical damage. If you remove the stress, then you reduce the muscle tension and relieve the Hurt. Sometimes when you use The Method to change a pain, inadvertently you can change underlying emotional Issues. It will never hurt to use The Method to try to reduce your symptoms.

Here is a sample of physical ailments and chronic illnesses for which partial or complete success has been obtained by addressing stress and remembered painful symptoms using The Method.

Allergies ✓	Morning sickness
Arthritis	Multiple sclerosis
Asthma	Muscle tightness
Back pain	Numbness in the fingers
Bee stings	PMS
Body sores	Poor coordination
Cancer	Psoriasis .
Carpal tunnel syndrome	Rashes
Chronic fatigue syndrome	Sexual dysfunctions
Constipation	Stiff neck and shoulders
Eyesight ✓	Stomach aches
Headaches	Sweating
Insomnia	Tooth aches
Irritable bowel syndrome	Trembling
Itching eyes	Ulcerative colitis
Joint pains	Urination problems
Lupus	

(After Craig and Fowlie, 1995)

Innerself Healing

A part of your personality is always alert and present in all your activities and experiences. This is your subconscious. I call this part your Innerself. The Innerself is like a sleeping resource. Most of us use it only for insight and problem solving. In the last 20 years, it has become increasingly obvious to many that the Innerself can participate in change processes. The Method is one of the change techniques that can be learned by the Innerself. Once learned, the Innerself can use it to change the emotions of negative beliefs, experiences or memories as they occur. As you read this book, your Innerself will pay close attention and remember everything you read. Once learned, the Innerself can mimic The Method, resolve problems that get in the way of change, and do the change process.

The final chapter will reveal additional resources to your Innerself. These resources will increase the ease, the independence and safety of the Innerself change processes.

The next chapter will give you a brief overview, like a glossary, of the concepts used in teaching The Method. It will briefly describe the five steps to do The Method and give an overview of several other significant chapters that are needed to ensure success.

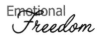

Chapter 2

Coming to Terms:
A Glossary of Chapter
Contents and Other Things

You have to know the concepts you're dealing with before you can start learning how to remove emotional pain from your life. This chapter serves up a glossary of key words you'll frequently find in this book. In later chapters, the book will define these terms in full. You'll also find each step of The Method spelled out several times and in different ways, so that when you reach the end you'll know how to use The Method to free yourself from painful emotions.

Changing Hurt

Hurt!! Hurt is a simple term I use to represent our anxiety, pain, fear, emotions, terror, aches and tension, and so forth. Hurt is the emotion you feel when you think of a painful Issue. You can have many disruptive Issues that can interfere with your ability to fully enjoy life. It is Hurt that is connected to a disruptive Issue that gives you problems. Whatever the Hurt, The Method changes the Issue so that it is no longer a problem. When you no longer have the disruptive Issue, you will feel better. Usually, we don't think about changing the Hurt, either because we are so used to the Hurt or because it fails to occur to us that our Hurt can be changed. But after reading this book and practicing The Method on small Issues to build your confidence, you can try it on anything and everything.

A Brief Overview

The words in **bold** are used repeatedly in this book. These definitions are very brief. Don't worry, they are explained in more detail below.

    Hurt is the term used to represent your painful emotions.

    An **Issue** is a problem, belief, emotion or pain that bothers you.

Aspects are different features of an Issue.

The **Affirmation** removes barriers to change by using a Saying and a Phrase.

The **Saying** is a positive, self-accepting statement in the Affirmation.

The **Phrase** is a two or three-word summary of the Hurt that is experienced with an Issue or Aspect.

The **Sequence** and **9-Gamut** are exercises that you will do, including tapping on acupressure points. These exercises change the Hurt of an Issue to neutral or positive emotions.

The Method includes the Affirmation, the Sequence, the 9-Gamut and the Sequence again. You will do these activities one after the other.

In the following chapters you will learn, with detailed descriptions, pictures and examples, the five skills needed to do The Method. You will learn:

1. How to Identify an Issue, the Aspects of an Issue, and how to make up Phrases.
2. How to do the Affirmation and the Modified Affirmation. Both have a Saying and a Phrase.
3. How to construct and do the Sequence by tapping on the 12 acupressure points.
4. How to do the 9-Gamut by tapping on a point while doing an exercise.
5. Just in case, how to Troubleshoot and eliminate other barriers to removing Hurt.

With these skills, you can use The Method to painlessly remove the Hurt from Issues. The Method consists of doing the Affirmation to remove a common barrier to change and then doing the Sequence, the 9-Gamut and the Sequence again to change the Hurt connected to an Issue. The Phrase is repeated at each tapping point. The Method is done a number of times until the experience of Hurt connected to an Issue is reduced or eliminated.

Aspects are different features of an Issue. By doing The Method with each Aspect of an Issue, the Issue is changed. When all Aspects have been changed by The Method, the experience of Hurt connected to an Issue is gone or reduced to an appropriate level. It may never return. If it does, do The Method on it.

Sometimes there may be a more complex barrier preventing change. If the Hurt does not change, you will have the Troubleshooting skills to be able to remove the barrier and obtain the change you want.

An Example Using The Method With a Height Phobia

Here is a brief run-through of The Method. If you have a height phobia, it is an Issue. Here is a description of the use of The Method to change the Hurt connected to an Issue. Issues can have Aspects. An Aspect of a height phobia might be the thought, "When I'm on a ladder, I am afraid." Each Aspect is given a short Phrase that describes the emotion of the Aspect. Here is an example of an Issue with two Aspects, each with its own Phrase:

Issue	Aspect	Phrase
Height phobia	When I'm on a ladder, I am afraid.	Fear of height
	I'm afraid I'll hurt myself if I fall.	Fear of injury

The Affirmation is a Saying and the Phrase. The Saying is a positive statement of self-acceptance. It is followed by the Phrase that describes the emotion of the Issue or Aspect. Here is an example of an Affirmation with a Saying and Phrase:

———————— **Saying** ——————— — **Phrase** —
"I accept myself even though I have a Fear of height."

The Affirmation is said three times, while rubbing a sore spot on your chest. It is said before you do the Sequence. The Sequence involves tapping on 12 acupressure points while saying the Phrase "Fear of height" out loud at each point. Then you do the 9-Gamut while thinking about the Phrase. The 9-Gamut consists of constantly tapping on an acupressure point on the back of your hand while doing six eye movements, and humming, counting and humming again. Then the Sequence is repeated the same way as before. You use The Method – the Affirmation, the Sequence, the 9-Gamut and the Sequence – as many times as necessary until the Hurt is gone. This all will be described later in further detail.

How It Works: Two Theories

The first theory is based upon the assumption that our body has a number of energy fields that flow on unique paths that are called meridians. Acupressure points are important points on the meridians. When we have an Issue, the Hurt is caused by the body's energy system being out of balance (Callahan, 1991). When you think of an Issue and tap on the acupressure points of the meridians associated with that Issue, the energy system associated with that Issue becomes balanced. Subsequently, when we think of the Issue, the Issue no longer elicits an emotional response.

The second theory is based on the assumptions that an Issue is associated with a number of major neural pathways, corresponding to what some people call meridians, and that sensory stimulation causes a memory process (Flint, in press, 94, 97). Again, by tapping on the acupressure points on the meridians, one is capable of stimulating those major neural pathways and, most important, of activating a memory process that causes change. This memory process that causes change is a memory process that effectively exchanges the current emotions for the emotions previously learned and associated with the Issue.

Here's how it works. The negative beliefs, flashbacks, pictures and movies that we call Issues consist of memories of experience and emotions. Interestingly, it appears that our brain distinguishes between memories of experience and memories of emotion and handles them differently. To distinguish between memories of experience and memories of emotion, I'll call memories of trauma emotion "Hurt" packets. Hurt packets, then, are connected to the meridians and other neural aspects associated with an Issue at the time of the trauma. When you actively think of an Issue, the

Hurt packets cause you to feel the emotions that were experienced during the trauma. On the other hand, when you are in a safe situation, you are usually experiencing neutral or positive emotions.

There is a memory packet that represents the emotional experience of a safe situation. Let's call it a "comfort" packet. Now, during the change process there are comfort packets that represent the emotions related to our present experience in the safe situation. Hurt memory packets, remember, are learned and/or attached to the meridians at the time of trauma. Therefore, when we tap on the acupressure points, which stimulates the memory process, we cause some number of comfort packets to replace the Hurt packets attached to the meridians associated with the Issue. Hence, when we stimulate the memory process by doing The Method with all the tapping, the experience of Hurt is gradually reduced as the Hurt packets connected to the Issue are replaced by comfort packets. In this way the pain of an Issue can be eliminated.

Selecting and Analyzing Issues

Selecting the Issues you want to change is easy, but sometimes Issues are complicated. They can have a number of Aspects that are associated with them. Big Issues can have many Aspects. Sometimes all the Aspects have to be changed before you notice a change in the big Issue. To make it easier for you, many Issues and Aspects are listed in Appendix I to help you find the Issues and their related Aspects.

It is very important to build trust in the power of The Method. This trust will give you the confidence to use the persistence that may be needed to overcome any barriers to change. To build confidence, you must begin by carefully selecting Issues that are easy to change, such as simple phobias rather than complicated Issues like addictions, compulsions or depression. So a series of small Issues, successfully changed, will build your confidence in The Method. With confidence, you will have the patience and persistence to successfully change any big Issue by Troubleshooting and overcoming its complexity.

Aspects

There may be more than one Aspect related to the Issue, the source of your Hurt. As you saw earlier, the height phobia had two Aspects: "When I am on a ladder, I am afraid" and "I'm afraid I will hurt myself if I fall." Whenever you find an Issue to change, it is important that you look for the related Aspects – the beliefs, emotions, pictures or sounds. When changing an Issue, The Method is used with each Aspect of the Issue. Turn to Appendix I and look for height phobia and other Issues and their Aspects.   ₽.1 ⌐

The Phrase

The Hurt related to each Aspect can be named with one or more words. For example, with the Aspect "I'm afraid I'll hurt myself," the Phrase would be "Fear of injury." You'll make a Phrase for each Aspect. When the first application of The Method does not eliminate the Hurt, add the word "remaining" to the Phrase and use this in the Modified Affirmation, for example, "The remaining fear of injury."

The Affirmation

The Affirmation is the first step in The Method. The Affirmation is made up of a Saying and a Phrase. The Saying sets a positive tone in your experience when you think of the negative Issue. The Phrase keeps the memory of the Issue in your experience. Here is an example of an Affirmation:

——————— **Saying** ——————— — **Phrase** —
"I accept myself even though I have this fear of injury."

The Modified Affirmation

When the Hurt does not decrease after doing The Method one or two times, you do the Modified Affirmation. This is just like the Affirmation, but the Saying and Phrase are modified to acknowledge the remaining Hurt. Notice the words in **bold**. The word "**remaining**" is added to the Phrase. The words in bold are said with emphasis. Here is an example of a Modified Affirmation:

———————— **Saying** ————————
"I accept myself even though I **still** have **some**

———— **Phrase** ————
remaining fear of injury."

The Sequence

By tapping on the 12 acupressure points, the Hurt is changed. You repeat the Phase out loud while tapping on each point to keep the memory of the Hurt in your experience, namely "Fear of injury" or "Remaining fear of injury." This will be explained in detail later.

The 9-Gamut

Hurt is sometimes connected with the eye positions, eye movements, or shifting brain activity that occurred during a trauma. You do the 9-Gamut in the following way. While tapping on the back of your hand, you move your eyes to different positions and hum (right brain) and count (left brain) to stimulate neural activity that might be associated with the memory of the Issue. The 9-Gamut addresses eight neural Aspects that can be associated with an Issue. By doing the 9-Gamut, you change the Hurt connected to one or more of these neural Aspects of your painful memory. The 9-Gamut will be explained in more detail later.

The Experiment

Although there is no question that The Method will work most of the time, the Experiment is just a way to convince you that The Method is effective for you. You will be scoring the change after each time you do The Method. The Score is a measure of how much it Hurts right now, when you think of the Issue or Aspect. For simplicity, you will be setting the starting Score for the Hurt of all Issues or Aspects to 10. No Hurt at all is 0. Scoring the Hurt is necessary so you can tell when the Hurt is changing, that is, getting less, or not changing – staying the same. When the Score of the Hurt doesn't change after doing The Method, start Troubleshooting. With some Issues, it is desirable to have some remaining Hurt with a Score of 1 or 2, namely with fear of heights or fear of water, and so forth. The Experiment, then, is a way to prove to yourself that you can use The Method to move the Score of some Issue or Aspect from a Score of 10 to a score of 0.

Troubleshooting the Barriers: How to Remove Them

When Hurt doesn't change, the change is stopped by a barrier. Barriers are a form of disorganization of the brain caused by memories related to an Issue, or some brain condition. The disorganization stops the change process. The Affirmation is done to make sure there are no memory-related barriers. However, there are many other conditions of the body that can cause brain disorganization and stop the change process. You will learn a number of corrections you can do to remove these barriers. Most are easy. Some are easier than others. You don't have to do them all at once. You select one or two corrections from the list and do The Method to see if it works. When it works, you are done. The corrections are given in the order in which you should try them. They are explained later in detail.

The corrections for removing barriers are the following: Use the Modified Affirmation, eliminate Shortcuts, increase your emphasis, correct brain polarity, drink 8 ounces of water, ask a friend to be a witness, review the Issue, move to different places, take a water-only shower, clear problematic food from your system, reduce the intake of toxic foods, eliminate some food barriers, or set up a schedule to do The Method. Be familiar with these corrections in case you discover a barrier.

Putting It All Together

When you want to change an Issue, your first task is to break the Issue down into as many Aspects as necessary. Write down a description of each Aspect and develop a Phrase that briefly describes the emotion or content of the Aspect. You will change each Aspect, one at a time. For each Aspect, set the Score of the Hurt to 10 and do The Method – the Affirmation, Sequence, 9-Gamut, and the Sequence again. After doing The Method, reassess the Score by guessing what it is. Repeat The Method until the Score goes to 0. Troubleshoot if the Score stops going down. Sometimes it is appropriate to have the Score greater than 0 when the Hurt has a protective purpose. Repeat this process with each Aspect until the Issue is changed.

It's Safe With Everyone

The Method can be used with everyone, young and old. Because it is so safe, it can be freely shared with family, friends and co-workers. But don't forget common sense. Be sure to start off with easy Issues so the person doesn't get discouraged or put off. Try it on everything: old pain, chronic pain, headaches – anything that can be stated as an Issue. It can't hurt to try The Method with any Issue that is a problem.

**But remember, read and understand
the book before you try it.**

Chapter 3

Picking Your Target: Selecting Issues, Aspects And Phrases

Zeroing in on a painful Issue is the first step toward removing emotional pain from your life, but there may be more to it. You've got to examine your Issue and identify all the various features, or Aspects, attached to it. Aspects are simply beliefs, emotions or sensations related either to the Issue you're working on or to the situation or trauma that caused the Issue.

In Appendix I, there are sample Issues with Aspects and Phrases. This appendix will help you to identify your Issues and assist you in finding Aspects and making Phrases.

The Issues, Aspects and Phrases are organized in Appendix I in the following way:

Issue	Aspect	Phrase
Height phobia	I am afraid of heights.	Fear of height
	I am afraid I'll hurt myself if I fall.	Fear of injury

Take a look now at Appendix I to get an idea of the kinds of Issues you can change. Notice that the Phrase can address the Hurt or the situation that causes the Hurt, or both. Use whichever generates the most Hurt. See "Claustrophobia in car" for a good example.

Here is another example to show you how complex it can get. This Issue is likely to be more difficult than any Issue you will have. Usually there are only one or two Aspects linked to an Issue. This really complex Issue illustrates the importance of looking for all the Aspects associated with an Issue.

For example, if you were the victim of a store robbery, you might have many Aspects to deal with that were caused by this experience.

Here are a few:

Beliefs:	It's not safe to work.
	Someday I'll die in a store robbery.
	I should have done something.
	I am not competent.
Emotions:	I feel anxious in stores.
	I always have an anxious feeling.
	I feel guilty that I didn't prevent it.
	I feel terror when I am downtown.
	I am afraid of dying.
	I am afraid to go to work.
Sensations:	Sirens frighten me.
	His face pops into my thoughts.
	The store door alarm frightens me.

These are 13 possible Aspects that could be related to the robbery Issue. You would use The Method with each Aspect. It is important to change all the Aspects of an Issue, because they all have Hurt connected to them. For this store robbery Issue, you would begin with the Aspect with the least amount of Hurt and continue through the list, one by one, working up to the Aspect with the most amount of Hurt. Since all these Aspects are interconnected, changing one Aspect may change other Aspects.

When doing The Method, it is important to understand that sometimes the Hurt related to the Issue does not decline until many of the Aspects are changed. Some Aspects may have to be worked with before The Method will affect other Aspects. So don't be discouraged if your Issue has a number of Aspects and continues to be Hurtful. Just continue doing The Method on the various Aspects of your Issue until the Hurt goes to 0.

After reviewing Appendix I, if you found some Issues that apply to you, write them down on a photocopy of the Issues Work Sheet. (See page 19 or tear out on page 101) For each of your Issues, write down the Aspects that are meaningful to you. Add any other Issues that you want to change that are not in the Appendix. Then write down the Aspects that are appropriate for each of these other Issues. Now, scan through Appendix I to see if any other Aspects would be appropriate for any of your Issues. Be sure you have written a Phrase for each Issue or Aspect.

Now you are going to use the form to decide the order in which you are going to change Issues. You will arrange them in order from the Issue with the least amount of Hurt to the Issue with the most amount of Hurt. Suppose you have five Issues (see the example) Using the first column (Iss. No.), write a 1 next to the Issue with the least Hurt and a 5 next to the Issue with the most Hurt. Then assign 2, 3 and 4, to the Issues with increasing Hurt. Now, using the third column, do the same with the Aspects for each Issue. In Issue 5, there are four Aspects. Using column three (Asp. No.), assign the numbers 1 to 4 to the Aspects from least Hurt, 1, to most Hurt, 4 (see the example). Do the same for the two Aspects of Issue 1.

Here is a completed Issues Work Sheet:

Issues Work Sheet

Card

Iss. No.	Issue	Asp. No.	Aspect	Phrase
1	Spider	2	I am afraid of spiders.	My fears
		1	I am afraid of moving spiders.	Moving spiders
4	Heeadache	–	I have anxiety headaches.	Anxiety headache
5	Sex abuse	2	I am afraid of that man.	My fear
		3	I have flashbacks.	My flashbacks
		1	I am afraid of sex.	My sex fear
		4	I am afraid when I see his car.	My fear
3	Sadness	–	I always feel sad.	My sadness
2	Needles	–	I am afraid of needles.	Fear of needles

By the way, with physical symptoms you order and change the symptoms from the symptom with the most Hurt to the symptom with the least Hurt.

Example

You are looking through Appendix I. You see "Fear of dentists." You know that one. Write down "Fear of dentists." You look at the Aspects and see that two of the four Aspects listed are true for you. You can feel some Hurt when you think of those Aspects and the dentist's office. You write those two Aspects and Phrases on the Issues Work Sheet. See the example below.

You think of another Issue. The Issue is "Chronic anxiety." You get your Issues Work Sheet and write "Chronic anxiety" in the Issue column. Then you write a sentence in the Aspect column that labels the emotion or problem that you experience, such as "I always feel anxious." Finally, you write a few words in the Phrase column that clearly capture your Hurt or the problem. You write "My anxiety." In this case you could find only one Aspect.

Iss. No.	Issue	Asp. No.	Aspect	Phrase
2	Fear of dentists	2	I am afraid of feeling pain.	Fear of pain
		1	I am afraid of the grinding.	Grinding fear
1	Chronic anxiety	1	I always feel anxious.	My anxiety

You order your Issues. "Fear of dentists" feels more intense than "Chronic anxiety." With only two Issues, you write 2 in the Issues number column (Iss. No.) next to "Fear of dentists," because it is the most intense. You put a 1 next to "Chronic anxiety" in the same column because it is the least intense. Look at the Issues with more than one Aspect. In this case it is "Fear of dentists." You think that "Fear of pain" is more intense than "Fear of grinding," so you put a 1 in the Aspect number column (Asp. No.) next to "Fear of grinding," the least intense, and 2 in the same column next to "Fear of pain" because it is the most intense. Now you are ready to do The Method on your Issues and Aspects.

Issues Work Sheet

List each Issue, develop the Aspects, if any, and write down the Phrases. Then number the Issues and Aspects as described in the book. Remember, assign 1 to the least Hurt.

Iss. No.	Issue	Asp. No.	Aspect	Phrase
—	————	—	——————————	————
—	————	—	——————————	————
—	————	—	——————————	————
—	————	—	——————————	————
—	————	—	——————————	————
—	————	—	——————————	————
—	————	—	——————————	————
—	————	—	——————————	————
—	————	—	——————————	————
—	————	—	——————————	————
—	————	—	——————————	————
—	————	—	——————————	————
—	————	—	——————————	————
—	————	—	——————————	————
—	————	—	——————————	————
—	————	—	——————————	————
—	————	—	——————————	————
—	————	—	——————————	————
—	————	—	——————————	————
—	————	—	——————————	————
—	————	—	——————————	————
—	————	—	——————————	————
—	————	—	——————————	————
—	————	—	——————————	————
—	————	—	——————————	————
—	————	—	——————————	————
—	————	—	——————————	————
—	————	—	——————————	————
—	————	—	——————————	————
—	————	—	——————————	————

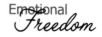

Chapter 4

Crashing the Barriers: Creating Affirmations

Barriers can stop change if you let them. Don't. The Method uses Affirmations and tapping to help you blast through those barriers on your road to an emotionally pain-free life.

Be sure you understand what a Phrase is. Look at the Phrases in the right column of the example on page 17. Notice that, in each case, the Phrase is just a brief way to clearly specify the Hurt or the situation giving rise to the Hurt. The Phrase is added to a Saying to form an Affirmation. Here is an example of a Saying and a Phrase:

_____ **Saying** _____
"I accept myself even though I have

____ **Phrase** ____
this fear of anxiety."

Try out some of the following Sayings to see which feels good to you.

   a. I deeply and profoundly accept myself even
       though I have the "Phrase."

   b. I love and accept myself and forgive myself for
       having the "Phrase."

   c. Even though I have the "Phrase," I deeply and
       completely accept myself.

   d. I accept myself even though I have the "Phrase."

   e. (For children) I'm okay even though I have the
       "Phrase."

For some, it is appropriate and helpful to add before the Affirmation, "With the help of God (Jesus), (Higher Power)," or simply imagine holding hands with Jesus while changing your Issue.

Here's how to do the Affirmation. Find a sore spot on the left side of your chest, about three inches down from the notch at the base of

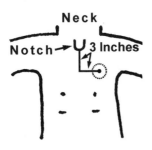

your throat in your chest plate and three inches to the left of midline (see figure). Use two fingers – the index finger and the middle finger. Search around for the sore spot. Rub in a circle on the sore spot to create some soreness while saying the Affirmation. While rubbing the sore spot, you will say the Affirmation three times at the beginning of The Method. Say it as if you believe it and mean it.

Sometimes the Affirmation or Saying doesn't feel true for you. Even if you don't believe the Affirmation, you say it as if you believe it to be true. Here are some examples of Affirmation statements with the Saying and the Phrase (**bold**):

"I accept myself even though I have **fear of heights**."

"Even though I **fear public speaking**, I deeply and completely accept myself."

Pick a Saying from the examples on page 20. Use a practice Phrase like "This Issue," and repeat the Affirmation with each of the example Sayings until you feel comfortable with one of the Sayings. Now, practice. Repeat the Affirmation out loud five to ten times while rubbing on the sore spot. Yes, it is important to **say it out loud.** Be sure to try different Sayings to see which feels the most comfortable to you.

Example

You have identified an Issue, "Chronic anxiety." You made an Affirmation by joining a Saying with a Phrase. The Affirmation is the first part of The Method. You carefully find a sore spot on your chest and start rubbing it, making it sore. You say the following Affirmation three times out loud while continuing to rub, "I accept myself even though I have my anxiety." Later, you will continue with the rest of The Method – the Sequence, 9-Gamut and the Sequence again.

Chapter 5

When Progress Sputters:
Boost the Power

Sometimes change will be stopped because barriers will pop up. At that point, you'll need the Modified Affirmation to give you the extra jolt you need to help you crash through those roadblocks. The modified variety is different from the straight Affirmation in two ways. First, by changing how the Saying is worded, you'll specifically focus on your acceptance of the remaining Hurt. Secondly, you'll add the word "remaining" before the Phrase in the Affirmation. You'll also add the word "remaining" before the Phrase as you are doing the Sequence and the 9-Gamut. Here is an example of the Modified Affirmation. You'll notice that it has a Saying and Phrase that emphasize the remaining Hurt associated with an Aspect.

—————————— **Saying** ——————————
"I accept myself even though I **still** have **some** of

—— **Phrase** ——
this **remaining** fear."

Notice the words **with bold letters**. Again, you will deliberately say these words in bold with emphasis and passion when you are saying the Modified Affirmation.

Try out your favorite Saying or others to see how they feel.

a. I deeply and profoundly accept myself even though I **still** have **some** of this **remaining** "Phrase."

b. I love and accept myself and forgive myself even though I **still** have **some** of this **remaining** "Phrase."

c. Even though I **still** have **some** of the **remaining** "Phrase," I deeply and completely accept myself.

d. I accept myself even though I **still** have **some** of the **remaining** "Phrase."

e. (For children) I'm okay even though I **still** have **some** of the **remaining** "Phrase."

Again, if it is appropriate for you, add before the Modified Affirmation, "With the help of God (Jesus), (Higher Power)," or, simply, imagine holding hands with Jesus while changing your Issue.

The Modified Affirmation is done in The Method just like the Affirmation described above, but with one exception. You get emotional and exaggerate the bold words in the Saying. Again, find the sore spot on your chest (see figure) and, while rubbing the sore spot in a circle, causing some pain, repeat the Modified Affirmation three times before you do the rest of The Method.

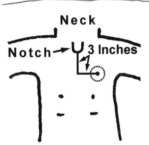

Try different Sayings to see which Saying feels most comfortable to you. Pick your Saying for the Modified Affirmation and a practice Phrase like "This remaining Issue." Repeat the Modified Affirmation **out loud** five to ten times while rubbing on the sore spot. Don't forget to exaggerate the words in bold. Again, it is important to say it out loud. Remember to add "remaining" to the Phrase.

Example

You have done The Method three times. Now, when you think "My anxiety," the Score feels like a 5 and not a 10. It feels about half as Hurtful as it did. The estimated Score came down to a 5 but did not change between the second and third use of The Method.

Remember that you use the Modified Affirmation in the first step of The Method when the score does not change. You say the following Modified Affirmation three times out loud while rubbing on the sore spot and exaggerating the words in **bold face**, "I accept myself even though I **still** have **some** of my **remaining** anxiety." You will later continue with the Sequence, the 9-Gamut and the Sequence again. Remember to say "My remaining anxiety" at each tapping point. Now, the Score went to 0 and you can feel no anxiety when you think of the Issue.

Chapter 6

Playing Taps:
Using Acupressure Points

To do the Sequence right, you've got to tap on 12 acupressure points to neutralize Hurt. How? Tap 5 to 7 times on each point. Say the Phrase out loud at each point to keep the Issue in your thoughts. When you're tapping, use these two tips: First, use the middle and index fingers to do the tapping. Second, learn to tap on the points in the exact order you'll read here. In order to get a good fix on each spot's location, as you read about each point, look carefully in a mirror to find that specific spot on your face or at the finger indicated.

Tap firmly, so you can hear the tap, but not so hard as to hurt yourself. With practice, the whole Sequence takes only 7 to 12 seconds. Start slowly and carefully at first so you locate the points correctly. Again, learn to tap with the index and middle fingers. It is easiest to learn to tap with both hands, but any variation with the left or right hand, or order of points, still works.

Here is the Sequence:

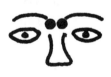

1. Eyebrow – While looking in a mirror, locate both spots at the beginning of the eyebrow and at the start of the bridge of the nose. Use both hands to tap on both sides. Be sure your spots are near the bridge of the nose. Tap 5 to 7 times on those spots.

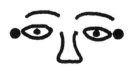

2. Outer Eye – Locate the spot on the bone next to the outside corner of the eye. Make sure you tap on the spot adjacent to the corner of the eye. Tap 5 to 7 times on those spots on the bone with both hands.

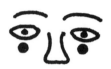

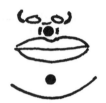

3. Under the Eye – Locate the spot on the top of the bone below the eye, directly below the pupil. Look in the mirror to see that you have located the right spots. Tap on those spots 5 to 7 times. Use both hands.

4. Under the Nose – Find the spot under the nose and tap with two fingers. Use only one hand.

5. Under the Lip – Find the spot under the lower lip on the indented area of the chin and tap.

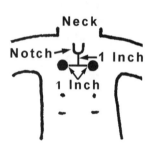

6. Collarbone – This point is a little more difficult to find. Locate the notch at the top of your breastbone or at the base of your throat (see figure). Put your fingers there and move them down 1 inch and over 1 inch on the right and left side of your chest. Look in a mirror and put your fingers on the collarbone spots. Be sure your fingers are **only 2 inches apart**. These are the collarbone spots. They are located on a depression under the joint of each collarbone. Tap these spots with both hands.

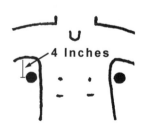

7. Under the Arm – Tap on a spot 4 inches under your underarms. If you are a female, tap on the bra line. If you are a male, tap on the spots level with the nipple. You can cross your arms to tap with your fingers or raise your arms and tap with your thumbs. Tap 5 to 7 times. Don't Giggle.

Now you will tap on four of your fingers and on the edge of your hand, one spot at a time. The figure of the left hand (see figure) shows the edge of your hand and which fingers you will tap: the thumb, index finger, middle finger and little finger. You will be tapping on each finger next to the base of the fingernail. This spot is on what I call the "inside of the finger." To get it right, put your left hand in front of you with your palm facing down. Find your index finger.

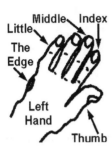

Here is a picture of the index finger of your left hand facing down so you can clearly identify the location of the base of the fingernail. The base of the fingernail is the cuticle (see figure). You will be tapping on the skin next to the base of the fingernail on the inside of the finger on the spot closest to your body.

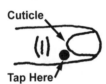

Carefully look at the pictures of the left hand fingers, palm facing down, and follow the instructions. Hold your left hand with your palm facing down.

8. **Thumb** – Find the spot on the inside of the thumb closest to the body. Tap on the skin next to the base of the thumbnail.

9. **Index Finger** – Find the spot on the inside of the index finger on the skin next to the base of the fingernail. Tap.

10. Middle Finger – Find the spot on the inside of the middle finger on the skin next to the base of the fingernail. Tap. After tapping, skip the ring finger and go to the little finger.

11. Little Finger – Find the spot on the inside of the little finger on the skin next to the base of the fingernail. Tap.

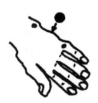

12. Karate Chop – Locate the spot on center of the soft skin on the outside edge of the hand, palm facing down. This spot is between the wrist knuckle and the little finger knuckle (see figure). Tap this spot 5 to 7 times.

Now to summarize. You will tap with two fingers on the following list of tapping points. Tap 5 to 7 times on each point. These are the 12 points of the Sequence.

 1. Eyebrow

 2. Outer Eye

 3. Under the Eye

 4. Under the Nose

 5. Under the Lip

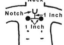 6. Collarbone

 7. Under the Arm

 8. Thumb

 9. Index Finger

 10. Middle Finger

 11. Little Finger

 12. Karate Chop

In order to learn the Sequence and to get used to doing it correctly, tap each point in the Sequence 5 to 7 times while saying a Phrase out loud at each tapping point. Look in a mirror to be sure you are tapping on the correct spots. You can gauge the number of taps with the time it takes to say the Phrase. Hey, you might get confused. It takes a little practice. If necessary, say the Phrase out loud and then tap 5 times on the point. If you tap more than 5 times, it's okay, it only takes longer. Practice the Sequence 5 to 10 times. But, before doing it, pause for a moment and say the following statement to yourself. "All the barriers that I may have to change are changing now" (T. Fleming, personal communication, September 24, 1998). Use the Phrase "My barriers" while practicing. The more you practice the easier it gets. Check to see that you are tapping on the correct spots.

Again, after using the Modified Affirmation, remember to say "remaining" with the Phrase at each tapping point in the Sequence, for example, "This **remaining** fear."

Example

You have the Issue of "Chronic anxiety" and write down the Phrase "My anxiety." The Method consists of the Affirmation, the Sequence, and the 9-Gamut, followed by the Sequence again. The Affirmation is the first part of The Method. You would say the following Affirmation out loud three times while rubbing on the sore spot: "I accept myself even though I have my anxiety." Then you do the first Sequence by tapping 5 to 7 times on each of the 12 acupressure points of the Sequence. You say "My anxiety" out loud at each point tapped. You do the 9-Gamut and then you do the Sequence again.

Chapter 7

Taking a Side Trip:
The 9-Gamut

Sometimes you must take a side trip to get where you're going. In The Method, that's the 9-Gamut. To do it, tap very fast on the back of your hand while doing the

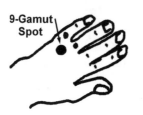

exercises in this chapter. You'll need some practice, because at first you'll feel awkward, as though you were rubbing your tummy and your head at the same time. To get started, on the back of either hand find the spot that is a half inch back from both the knuckle of the ring and little finger (see figure). Just tap at least 3 to 5 times per second repeatedly and firmly. Try tapping rapidly for five seconds and count the number of taps. While tapping, do the exercises below at the same time.

While **tapping rapidly** and holding your **head upright**, do the following:

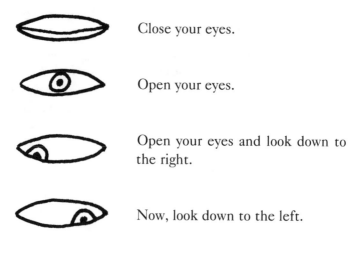

Close your eyes.

Open your eyes.

Open your eyes and look down to the right.

Now, look down to the left.

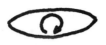

Whirl your eyes in a wide circle in one direction, then . . .

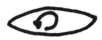

Whirl your eyes in a wide circle in the other direction.

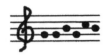

Hum a few notes, like "Happy Birthday to You" or some other tune. It is important to hum 4 or 5 different notes **out loud**.

Say: "1, 2, 3, 4, 5"

Count out loud, "One, two, three, four, five."

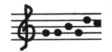

Hum a few notes, "Happy Birthday" or some other tune. Remember, hum 4 or 5 different notes **out loud**.

9-Gamut Spot

Now to summarize. You will tap repeatedly with two fingers on the 9-Gamut spot and do the following exercises with your eyes and your voice:

  Close your eyes

  Open your eyes

  Open, look down to the right

  Look down to the left

  Circle your eyes one way

  Circle your eyes the other way

  Hum a tune out loud

Say: "1, 2, 3, 4, 5" Count from 1 to 5 out loud

Hum a tune again out loud

You have just completed the 9-Gamut. Practice the 9-Gamut until you can do it without thinking. When you can do that, practice doing the 9-Gamut while holding or saying the Phrase in your thoughts. Just as it is important to say the Phrase with each tapping point on the Sequence, it is important to hold the Phrase in your thoughts while you are doing the 9-Gamut. Of course, it's not easy when you are tapping, moving your eyes, humming, and counting. Just say the Phrase out loud when you start the 9-Gamut and intend to hold the Phrase in your thoughts and you will do fine.

While holding the Phrase in your thoughts, practice doing the 9-Gamut until you can do it easily in 5 to 10 seconds. Later, you will assemble the Affirmation, the Sequence and the 9-Gamut into The Method. Look at Appendix II. Wallet-sized reminders for the Sequence and the 9-Gamut are on a page that you can photocopy.

Example

You notice you have some anxiety. You whip out your wallet-sized reminders and get ready to do The Method. You set the Score to 10 and, referring to the reminder, do the Affirmation and complete the first Sequence. You remembered to say "My anxiety" **out loud** at each tapping point. The 9-Gamut is done after doing the first Sequence. You think "My anxiety" and do the 9-Gamut by tapping repeatedly on the spot on the back of your hand. While tapping repeatedly and checking your reminder, you look straight ahead, close your eyes, open your eyes, look down to the right, look down to the left, circle your eyes one way all the way around, circle your eyes the other way, hum a few bars of "Happy Birthday," count "1, 2, 3, 4, 5" and hum a few bars of "Happy Birthday" again. You made sure to hum and count **out loud**. After doing the 9-Gamut, you tap 5 to 7 times on each of the 12 points of the Sequence, again saying "My anxiety" **out loud** at each tapping point. You have just completed The Method. Now reassess the Score.

Chapter 8

Skepticism Antidote:
The Three Experimental Steps

You have every right to be skeptical. For all you skeptics, though, you should know that, according to Gary Craig, The Method results in noticeable improvement in 50 to 80 percent of those who use it, depending on their level of expertise. "Yeah, right," you'll be thinking. Well, prove it to yourself by experimenting. When you try something new, you're running a private experiment to see if it works. Everything you do to change your Issues is also an experiment. So do a series of experiments. If they work, you'll develop more confidence in The Method – confidence you'll need for more difficult Issues. You'll boost your success with The Method considerably if you'll just perform the following three steps:

1. **Find the Aspects** – After you have found a problem or Issue, you have to carefully explore the Issue to uncover all the related Aspects. If you miss a significant Aspect of your Issue, there is some possibility that The Method will not change the Issue. To successfully change Issues, all the Aspects have to be found and changed. Once you have all the Aspects listed, do The Method with the Aspect with the least Hurt and, one by one, work up to the Aspect with the most Hurt. Notice in Appendix I that it is not uncommon to find only one Aspect for an Issue.

2. **Score the Progress** – The Score is a measure of how intensely a Hurt is felt. It is very important to use a scoring system during the process. This means that you estimate the Score of the Hurt before you start and after each time you do The Method. You will want to know that the Score is going down and that The Method is working. Also, and most important, when the Score doesn't change you will have to Troubleshoot.

There are many ways to have a scoring system. Let's keep it simple. Let's have 10 be the measure of the initial Hurt of all Issues or Aspects that you'll be working with. A score of 10 can be a big Hurt or little Hurt. Either way, 10 represents the starting Hurt. You will want to see the Hurt decrease when you do The Method. People who don't like numbers can draw a line with 10 or high on one end and 0 or none on the other. After they do The Method, they can put a mark on the line to show where they Score the Hurt. Kids can have a range of faces from a sad face to a happy face to help them Score the changes in their Issue or Aspect.

KIDS

Here's how to experience the starting intensity of Hurt or emotion linked to your Issue or Aspect. If you already know the Hurt of the Issue is very intense and also know the feeling, don't bother to do this. That high intensity is Scored a 10. If you don't know the feeling and want to experience the intensity of the starting Hurt, think of the Issue or say the Phrase to yourself out loud. The intensity of the emotion that you now feel is the starting intensity that you call a 10. Now you know what the score of 10 feels like. It's the starting Hurt. You all know when the Score is 0. There is absolutely no Hurt. It's like the emotional intensity you feel when you look at a kitchen cupboard. Every time you do The Method on an Issue, you expect the Score to change. The starting score for an Issue is 10, and the final score is 0. After each time you do The Method, you estimate or guess the new Score. When the Hurt doesn't change, the score doesn't change. If it changes, you guess. A guess is not right or wrong, it's just a guess. You guess the Score after doing The Method to keep track of the changes. Hey, remember that it is only a guess and you just want to keep a record of the change in the intensity of Hurt. As you do The Method, the Score should change from 10 to 0.

There is a good reason to Score the change in Hurt. You have to know when the effect of The Method has stopped – in other words, when it is not working. If the Score gets stuck between 10 and 0 and doesn't change, then you turn to chapter ten, the Troubleshooting chapter. You Troubleshoot until you discover the barrier that stopped the change. You do this through the process of elimination. There are 13 corrections to use to eliminate barriers. By correcting for potential barriers, one correction at a time, you will eventually find the barrier that prevented the change, and the Score will begin to decrease again. This will be described later in greater detail.

3. **Bring the Score to 0** – Continue using The Method until there is no more Hurt connected to the Issue or Aspect. Some people stop too soon and believe The Method didn't work. By feeling and Scoring the Hurt and experiencing the changes, these people will be more likely to reduce their Hurt to 0. Remember, when the Score stops changing, turn immediately to chapter ten on Troubleshooting. Use patience and persistence to find the correction for the barrier.

To build your confidence in The Method, do the Experiment by carefully selecting Issues and Aspects with low intensity, setting the initial Score before you start, obtaining a score after each time you do The Method, and, by repeating The Method, reduce the Score to 0. If you have barriers, Troubleshoot with patience and persistence.

Example

You start the Experiment by setting the Score. Think of the Phrase "My anxiety" to experience the intensity of the Hurt. Assign this feeling a Score of 10. You do The Method repeatedly. Each time, after doing The Method, you experience the Hurt in your own way or by thinking "My anxiety." Estimate the Score in comparison to the 10, the starting intensity, and 0, no Hurt. You watch the Score decrease to 0 after doing The Method a number of times. In this way, you can prove to yourself that The Method will work.

If the Score doesn't go to 0, you do the other part of the Experiment, which is to Troubleshoot. By Troubleshooting, you can discover the correction for the barrier that keeps the Score from decreasing. With patience and persistence, and Troubleshooting, you can move the Score to 0, again proving to yourself that The Method works for you. With successful Experiments, you gain confidence in using The Method.

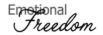
Chapter 9

Less Is More:
Why Sometimes a Shortcut Works

Hey!! Sometimes Shortcuts work – you can drop out parts of The Method and get change. But don't read this chapter until you believe The Method really does change your Issues and can get rid of your Hurt. If you don't, then trying Shortcuts only means you're shortchanging the process. The Method may not work, and you'll get discouraged. If you do believe the process works, then, when a Shortcut works, it will save you time and you can still make changes. Here's the test: If you can easily Troubleshoot barriers, then you're ready to try Shortcuts.

Although the complete Method is most thorough in reducing Hurt and is pretty fast, there are Shortcuts that can be taken when using The Method. Be aware that if The Method does not work with a Shortcut, then the Shortcut should be eliminated. In this case, The Method with no Shortcuts should be used again to obtain its full effectiveness.

The Method consists of the Affirmation, the Sequence, the 9-Gamut, and the Sequence again. Here are the four ways to shorten The Method:

1. **Shorten the Sequence** – Do the first seven tapping points as follows:

     1. Eyebrow
     2. Outer Eye
     3. Under the Eye
     4. Under the Nose

     5. Under the Lip
     6. Collarbone
     7. Under the Arm

    Tapping on these points usually obtains the desired results, so after you have confidence in The Method, you might routinely use this Shortcut if you choose.

2. **Leave out the Affirmation** – The Affirmation is necessary only about 40 percent of the time. Do the Sequence, 9-Gamut and the Sequence without the Affirmation. However, if the Score does not decrease from 10 to 8, put the Affirmation back into The Method. Also, if The Method works, but later the Score does not decrease after two applications, put the Affirmation or the Modified Affirmation back into The Method.

3. **Leave out the 9-Gamut** – Sometimes the 9-Gamut can be left out. It will really be necessary only about 30 percent of the time. If the Score doesn't decrease after a few applications, put the 9-Gamut back in.

4. **Use the most effective tapping point** – Some people find one tapping point is most effective in changing a pain or a symptom. With chronic symptoms, it may be convenient just to tap on this one point.

In most cases, the full Method is the most effective way to reduce the Hurt. Remember, if you try a Shortcut and The Method doesn't work, replace the steps in The Method that you have removed.

Example

You have identified an Issue, "Chronic anxiety," and set the starting Score to 10. You get the feeling of the starting intensity of the Issue by thinking about the Issue or saying the Phrase, "My anxiety." You want to use a Shortcut. You do The Method and leave out the Affirmation and the 9-Gamut to save a little time. This means that you just do the Sequence repeatedly, checking the Score each time, until the Score goes to 0. You remember to say "My anxiety" out loud at each tapping point. If it doesn't work to reduce the Score to 0, you eliminate the Shortcuts and do The Method again. If the Score goes to 0, you are done. If the Score doesn't change, you use patience and persistence, and start Troubleshooting.

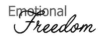

Chapter 10

When You've Been Derailed: How to Get Back on Track

If you aren't making progress and The Method doesn't work, it's easy to get discouraged and lose interest. Troubleshooting is too important to pass over. Remember, if you can make a series of small changes, your confidence will grow. That means that you don't use Shortcuts or tackle big Issues until you're confident and The Method has worked for you a couple of times. In this chapter, you'll get a plan to systematically get your progress moving again. Once you learn this Troubleshooting format, you won't get discouraged if The Method temporarily stops working.

Anyone who uses The Method may have times when Issues get stuck; the Score does not change. When this happens, a barrier is blocking the change process. Identifying the correction for the barrier is a process of trial and error. The following 13 corrections are listed in the order in which you should try them. It's simple. You try one correction and do The Method without Shortcuts. If the Score does not go down, you try the next correction. You continue this strategy, trying one correction after the other, until the Score goes down.

Persistence is the key. As in any project that runs into difficulties, persistence is needed to complete the project successfully. Persistence means you keep Troubleshooting. Because there are a number of conditions that can serve as barriers to change, persistence is necessary to complete the trial-and-error process needed to change the Hurt successfully.

Brief descriptions of the corrections for barriers are presented here in the order in which you should try them. Skipping around is also acceptable, especially when you have an idea about what the barrier could be. Review the corrections, so you know what they are. The following list, showing what you have to do for each of the 13 corrections, is given to show you how easy it is to Troubleshoot. Most corrections are simple to do. These will all be explained in more detail on the following pages. Remember, you can Troubleshoot by trying the corrections in the order given below.

Here are the most common corrections that are easy to do:
1. Use the Modified Affirmation – It's easy.
2. Eliminate Shortcuts – Do The Method without Shortcuts.
3. Increase your emphasis – Use passion with the Affirmation and tapping.
4. Brain polarity – Don't ask how or why; it just takes three seconds to do.
5. Drink 8 ounces of water – Time it, five seconds.

These corrections are slightly more difficult:
6. Ask a friend to be a witness – A simple assertion.
7. Review the Issue – Look for more Aspects or related Issues.
8. Move to different places – Easy to do with little effort.
9. Water-only shower – Forget soap and scrub. Do The Method in the buff.

The most intense corrections require more patience and persistence:
10. Clear the body – Watch what you eat and wait for three days.
11. Reduce intake – Eat less of some food items and wait three days.
12. Common food barriers – This is demanding, but not impossible.

Here is the correction for addictions and pervasive problems:
13. Scheduling The Method – This is like taking pills on a schedule.

Remember, when The Method is working, the Score of the Hurt changes. When there is no change in the Score, you have a barrier. The following corrections are the most common:

1. **Modified Affirmation** – If you have forgotten to do the Modified Affirmation, try The Method again with the Modified Affirmation. The Affirmation is the first part of The Method and is specifically used to correct barriers frequently found with Issues. Sometimes it is necessary to use the Modified Affirmation with every application of The Method. In this case, the Score will sometimes go down 1 point at a time.

2. **Eliminate Shortcuts** – If you have been taking Shortcuts, stop taking them. Use the whole Method with all 12 points, and the 9-Gamut to see if the Hurt can be changed. Be sure to include the Affirmation or the Modified Affirmation.

3. **Increase Your Emphasis** – Try all the following suggestions, from a to e, at the same time, before doing anything else.
   a. Even if you don't believe it, say the Affirmation or Modified Affirmation with increased emphasis, with conviction and passion.
   b. Be sure to say the Phrase out loud at each tapping point.
   c. Use "remaining" before the Phrase if appropriate.
   d. Make sure you are tapping on the correct spots.
   e. Tap a little harder so you can hear the tap. Don't bruise yourself.

4. **Brain Polarity** – This barrier is a condition that causes a form of brain disorganization that stops the change process. As 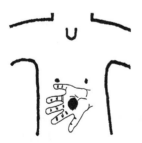 strange as it may seem, by placing the back of your hand on your chest (see figure), and then tapping on your palm 5 times, this barrier is corrected. Sometimes, if change is very slow, doing this correction before the Modified Affirmation will cause more rapid change.

5. **Drink Water** – This is an easy one. Drink 8 ounces of water and try The Method again.

If the previous corrections don't produce results, you may have to do the following, less common, corrections:

6. **Ask a Friend to Witness** – Do The Method in the presence of a friend. This public commitment reaffirms your intention to change the Hurt. If there is still no change, have your friend tap on the points. Having your friend tap the Sequences and the 9-Gamut can occasionally make the difference and result in change.

7. **Review the Issue** – Look for more Aspects of the Issue. If your Issue has a number of Aspects, attempting to change the Issue by using only one Aspect may not work. When the whole Method does not work to reduce the Score, look for other Aspects related to the Issue. Then use The Method on each Aspect. Often you may have to get more specific when describing an Issue. For example, with the Issue "I am afraid of water," the Aspects may be fear of having your head underwater, fear of suffocating, fear of water in the eyes, nose, ears, and so forth.

The following Troubleshooting approaches are corrections for barriers that occur less frequently. They have to do with your environment:

8. **Change Location** – We all have experienced a disturbance in our brain caused by the smell of perfume or industrial solvents. This is the first correction that deals with chemicals that may be causing a barrier. Move to another place – the kitchen, the bathroom, outside or elsewhere – to try The Method. If trying The Method in another place works, then some chemical or property of the environment may have been causing the barrier.

9. **A Water-only Shower** – Take a shower without using soap and scrub well with a wash cloth all over your body. You do this to remove all those chemicals off your body – chemicals

like deodorant, perfume, soap, shampoo and toothpaste, and
so forth. Try The Method in your birthday suit while
standing barefoot in the shower, the bathroom or elsewhere
in the house. If that doesn't work, stand on plastic wrap and
try it again. If this works, then something on your body, on
the floor or in your clothing was the problem.

The next barriers are food-related. Write down what you eat for a
number of days as you do the following problem-solving. It will
help you identify what food, if any, may be blocking The Method.

10. **Clear the Body** – Sometimes the source of the barrier may
    be caused by an unusual food that you ate. Wait a couple of
    days to let the source of the barrier pass out of your system,
    then try it again. This will work only if the food-related
    problem is not in your regular diet.

11. **Reduce Intake** – If you overeat some foods, they may cause
    a barrier. Foods like potatoes, carrots, peas, plums and others
    have chemicals that can cause a barrier if too much is eaten.
    Watch your diet to see if you are eating any foods excessively.
    Eliminate that food from your diet for several days and see if
    The Method works. If this doesn't work, look for other foods
    that might be the cause of the problem.

12. **Food Barriers** – If all else fails, look for allergies. Some
    people are allergic to the items listed below. These items,
    especially nicotine and caffeine, can sometimes cause barriers.
    Occasionally, one or more of these items must be eliminated
    from one's diet to get The Method to work. They don't have to
    be eliminated forever. They have to be removed just to use The
    Method. Foods and other items that are frequently found to
    cause barriers are the following:

Refined Sugar	Tea	Nicotine
Wheat	Pepper	Caffeine
Corn	Herbs	Alcohol

If some or all of these items are eliminated from your diet for a week, you have removed some of the most common allergy sources that can block change by inhibiting the effectiveness of The Method. Most likely, The Method will work without these substances in your body.

The following Troubleshooting approach is used routinely with addictions and chronic symptoms. It is usually the last resort in Troubleshooting, but can be used whenever you think it is appropriate, say, with an addiction, chronic symptom, or an obsession that is particularly entrenched. It can also be used before food barriers are investigated:

13. **Scheduling The Method** – Sometimes Issues are complex and you will have to set up a schedule. An example of the schedule is doing The Method three times on an Issue, five times throughout the day. The five times could be when you get up, at lunch time, at dinner time, in the evening and at bedtime. The number of times is flexible. Scheduling The Method is commonly used with depression, addictions and degenerative diseases. With addictions, it may be necessary to do The Method every half hour to bring the urge under control. It is also important to point out that just by doing the schedule on some general Issue, you can cause subtle, positive changes in your life without your awareness. A schedule requires dedication, but sometimes it is necessary. A form to organize your schedule is given on page 45. Here is an example of a schedule that is set up for nine repetitions per day.

Scheduling Form

Date	Schedule								
	8am	*10am*	*Noon*	*2pm*	*4pm*	*6pm*	*8pm*	*10pm*	*12pm*
6-11	✓	✓	✓	—	✓	✓	✓	✓	—
6-12	✓	✓	✓	✓	—	✓	✓	—	✓
6-13	✓	✓	✓	✓	✓	✓	✓	✓	✓
6-14	—	✓	✓	✓	✓	✓	✓	—	✓
6-15	✓	✓	✓	✓					

Most people will not have to deal with intense Troubleshooting activity. The Method will most likely eliminate or decrease Hurt from whatever Issue you want to change.

If you have persistently tried all these Troubleshooting approaches and The Method still does not work, don't give up. Look in Appendix V for resources to help you resolve the problem or change the Issue.

Example

You have an Issue, "Chronic anxiety." You experience the starting intensity and set the Score to 10. You do The Method without the Affirmation. You check the Score. You think "My anxiety," and notice no change from the starting intensity – that is, the Score is still 10 and did not change. Now you have to Troubleshoot to discover the barrier that is blocking change. You do this by the process of elimination. You start by eliminating the Shortcut (correction 2) and do The Method including the Affirmation. Again, the Score does not change. You select the first Troubleshooting option and do The Method with the Modified Affirmation(1). Again, no change. You use the third correction and do The Method with increased emphasis(3). Oh . . . no change. You do the correction for a brain polarity(4). Again, no change. You drink 8 ounces of water(5) and do The Method. Again, no change. You get your friend to witness your doing the tapping and have him do the tapping(6). Sigh . . . no change. Now, you review the Issue and look for other Aspects(7). You can't find any other Aspects, so you do The Method in different rooms, outside, and in the hot tub for the fun of it(8). Still no change. Continuing, you take a water-only shower(9), scrubbing with a clean washcloth and no soap. You try The Method standing in the shower and the Score reduces to 0. You found the barrier. There must have been a chemical on your body or in your clothes that caused the barrier. Your patience and persistence with Troubleshooting has changed the Issue. Your Experiment was successful and your confidence grows.

Scheduling Form

Write the activity or hour on the first line to remind you when to do
The Method. On the following lines, write the date, then put your
check mark under the scheduled time.

Date   **Schedule**

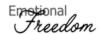

Chapter 11

Surveying the Landscape:
An Overview

This chapter is for you if you're interested in a thumbnail sketch of The Method. Using this summary can help you build your skills and make your using The Method even more effective.

1. Write down your Issues and Aspects, and, for each Aspect, make up a Phrase. Use a copy of the Issues Worksheet on page 19.

2. Obtain an Affirmation by selecting a Saying and adding a Phrase to it. Each Issue or Aspect has its own Phrase.

3. You perform an Experiment on each Issue or Aspect by feeling the Hurt and setting the Score to 10. The point of the Experiment is to reduce the Hurt to 0.

4. Then do The Method. The Method is the Affirmation, the Sequence, the 9-Gamut, followed by the Sequence again. Do the Affirmation 3 times; then do the Sequence, saying the Phrase out loud at each point; then, while holding the Phrase in your thoughts, do the 9-Gamut, and repeat the Sequence again, saying the Phrase out loud at each point. Check out Appendix II for a convenient summary of the points.

5. Assess the Score. If it is going down, Do The Method again. When it reaches a Score of 0, stop.

6. When you run into barriers that stop the Score from changing, start Troubleshooting. Continue doing The Method and Troubleshooting, if necessary, to obtain a Score of 0.

That's it. If you have any questions at this point, look in the index, read chapter two or read any other appropriate chapter to answer your questions. If you have no questions, you are ready to begin.

Doing The Method

If you haven't listed your Issues already, tear out page 101, photocopy the Issues Work Sheet on page 19, or take out a piece of paper and make your own Issues Work Sheet. List the Issues that you want to work on. Leave a number of lines after each Issue to list the Aspects. Look through Appendix I for additional help in finding other Issues you may have. If you find more Issues there, write down the Issue and any Aspects that cause you some Hurt or that you think are relevant to you. You can always read all the Aspects in Appendix I to get ideas for other Aspects. If you find only one Aspect, don't worry; sometimes an Issue has only one Aspect.

When you finish, your work sheet should look something this:

Iss. No.	Issue	Asp. No.	Aspect	Phrase
3	Anxiety		I am always anxious.	My anxiety
1	Height phobia	1	I am afraid of heights.	Fear of height
1		2	I'm afraid I'll hurt myself.	Fear of injury
2	Fear of dark		I am afraid of the dark.	Fear of dark
4	Sadness		I have sadness at bedtime.	That sadness

Now, you are going to use the Issues Work Sheet to determine the order in which you are going to change Issues. The example worksheet shows four Issues. We are going to order the four Issues from least Hurt (1) to most Hurt (4). Using the first column for the Issue Number (Iss. No.), write 1 next to the Issue with the least Hurt and a 4 next to the Issue with the most Hurt. Then assign the 2 and 3 to the remaining Issues from least Hurt, 2, to next most Hurt, 3. Using the third column for the Aspect Number (Asp. No.), do the same with the Aspects for each Issue. In this example, only Issue 1 has more than one Aspect. Using the Asp. No. column, assign 1 to the Aspect with the least Hurt and assign 2 to the Aspect with the most Hurt.

Now that you have your Issues and Aspects in order from least Hurt to most Hurt, you can start Experimenting. Take the Issue that has the least Hurt and do The Method on that Issue. If there is more than one Aspect, start with the least Hurtful Aspect and use The Method. If the Score decreases more than 2 units, repeat The Method using the Modified Affirmation. If the Score stays at 9 or 10 or is stuck somewhere between 1 and 10, even when using the Modified Affirmation, use the Troubleshooting options and persistence to eliminate the barrier. Troubleshoot and repeat The Method until the Score goes to 0.

Do The Method on all the Aspects belonging to each Issue. Remember, do the Issues from least Hurt to most Hurt. Do the same for the Aspects of an Issue, that is, from least Hurt to most Hurt.

When you have finished changing an Issue, there are two things you can do to be sure you have completed the job. First, carefully review the Issue and try to find any remaining Hurt that is still present. Second, describe the Issue in detail, to a friend, to see if any Hurt remains. Do The Method on any remaining Hurt. If the Hurt does not change, use persistence and Troubleshooting to discover why the Score doesn't reduce to 0. Sometimes a Score of 1 or 2 is an appropriate level of Hurt, that is, it is at a level that keeps you alert about something, for example, climbing tall ladders or swimming in the ocean.

If you still can't reduce your Hurt, turn to Appendix V to get some help.

Use Common Sense

This is a safe procedure, but sometimes the extreme trauma that disrupts people's lives is too great to be changed without some professional supervision. There are two circumstances where one has to be careful: First, when you are aware of severe trauma, and second, when you have forgotten traumatic memories that you don't remember as an adult. Here is what to do:

History of Severe Trauma – If you have a history of severe trauma, there is some chance that your life could be disrupted by sudden fear, pain or flashbacks, and so forth, by using The Method.

Please work with a therapist just in case you have some emotional upset. When you are doing The Method in your therapist's presence and the emotions start to increase, follow your therapist's direction or just continue doing The Method with no Shortcuts persistently and repeatedly until the emotions subside.

No Memory of a Traumatic History – If you have trauma and no memory for it, you may not have any clue that you have severe trauma in your history. If you can't remember your childhood, have blank spots in your experience, have two or more voices chattering in your thoughts or notice that things move around in your house mysteriously, then there is some chance that you have amnesic or dissociated memories. If you have any of these experiences, consult with a therapist. But suppose you don't have these experiences and you are not aware of any trauma. If you try The Method and your emotions start to sharply increase in intensity, stop and consult with a registered or licensed therapist.

See Appendix V for further help in finding a therapist.

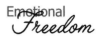
Chapter 12

Go with the Flow:
Learning from Charts

This chapter is for people who like flow charts and learn well from them. If that description doesn't fit you, then skip to the next chapter. It's not necessary to read a flow chart to benefit from The Method. If you like flow charts, this chart will describe all the decision points you can reach using The Method. The following information describes the flow chart on page 52.

As you read the following, trace the path in the flow chart.

The flow chart starts off by identifying the Issue and then the Aspects associated with the Issue. Next, for each Aspect, you develop Phrases for the Affirmation. Then you have the option to use Shortcuts. I don't advise this until you have more experience with The Method. Next, you assess the Hurt and set the Score to 10. Now you're ready to go. Do the Affirmation three times, then the Sequence, the 9-Gamut and the Sequence again. Don't forget to repeat the Phrase out loud at each tapping point and hold the Phrase in your thoughts while doing the 9-Gamut. Assess the Hurt and obtain a Score. Now, there are three possible outcomes:

1. **Slow/No Change** – The Score didn't change or changed only one point. In this case you go immediately to the Troubleshooting list. You can try the corrections one by one. After each correction, you enter the flow by doing the three Affirmations and continue. You will return to Troubleshooting if the Score does not change. If your have discovered other Aspects, then you start at the top. Notice the contents in the Troubleshooting box and the lines returning to The Method.

2. Partial Relief – The Score decreases by 2 or more points. This is partial relief. Do the Modified Affirmation three times and then do the Sequence, the 9-Gamut and the Sequence again. Remember that sometimes the Score will go down 1 point at a time. When this happens, try using both the Modified Affirmation and correction four for brain polarity (see page 40) when you do The Method. Follow the line in the flow chart.

3. Complete Relief – The Score goes to 0 or an adaptive level. Test the Issue by describing it in detail to a friend. If you find another Aspect or more Hurt, go back to the top of the flow chart. Of course, with no Hurt or Aspects, you are done. Notice the line in the flow chart.

So there it is. The whole flow chart pulling it all together. With or without the flow chart, if you understand The Method, you can change most of your Issues.

Flow Chart of The Method

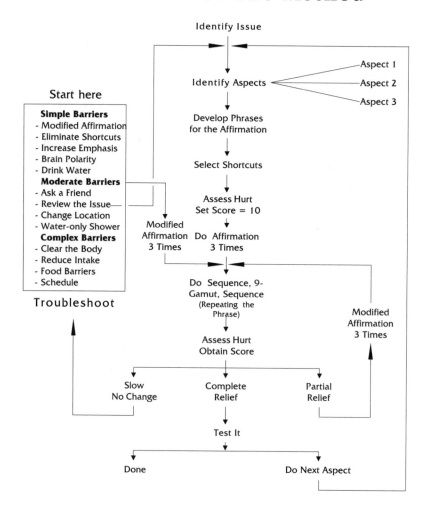

Identify Issue

Identify Aspects — Aspect 1
— Aspect 2
— Aspect 3

Start here

Simple Barriers
- Modified Affirmation
- Eliminate Shortcuts
- Increase Emphasis
- Brain Polarity
- Drink Water

Moderate Barriers
- Ask a Friend
- Review the Issue
- Change Location
- Water-only Shower

Complex Barriers
- Clear the Body
- Reduce Intake
- Food Barriers
- Schedule

Troubleshoot

Develop Phrases
for the Affirmation

Select Shortcuts

Assess Hurt
Set Score = 10

Modified
Affirmation   Do Affirmation
3 Times   3 Times

Do Sequence, 9-
Gamut, Sequence
(Repeating the
Phrase)

Assess Hurt
Obtain Score

Modified
Affirmation
3 Times

Slow   Complete   Partial
No Change   Relief   Relief

Test It

Done   Do Next Aspect

Chapter 13

Getting the Gunk Out: Changing the Oil and Cleaning the Carburetor

You know how much better it is for your car when you change the oil and clean the carburetor. The sludge buildup is gone, and the engine runs smoother and longer. Your experience of life is much the same. Painful thoughts can make your life run a lot rougher than it needs to. Using The Method, you can clean out your unwanted beliefs and traumatic memories by healing almost any negative experience. In this chapter, we will explain the difference between changing a belief and changing a traumatic memory.

To change a traumatic memory Issue, you will focus upon the memory or the Hurt when you do The Method to reduce the Hurt (see page 34). However, when changing a belief, you will focus on the truth of the negative belief when you use The Method to change the belief. It appears as if the Hurt connected to the belief – the memory of the statement of the belief, if you will – determines how true the belief is for you. When the Hurt is removed from the memory, the belief is no longer true for you and the belief or traumatic memory will no longer intrude on your thoughts. A description of how to use The Method to change beliefs will be given in this chapter.

You may have an unwanted or self-limiting belief that bothers you. If you do, you would probably want to change the belief because life would be more satisfying if you didn't have it. If the belief is "I'm not worthy of love," the first thing you would do is assess your experience of how true this belief is for you. Again, for simplicity, regardless of how true it is, you set the Score to 10. Ten is a measure of how true the belief is for you. The purpose of doing The Method with the belief is to change the Score for the belief to 0 – that is, change the belief so it is no longer true for you. To do this, you simply make up a Phrase, say, "Unworthy of love," to use when you are doing The Method. Now, do The Method remembering to say the Phrase out loud at each tapping point. Repeat The Method until the Score of belief shows that it is no longer true for you. By scoring the truth of the belief, you can tell if The Method is working or if there is a barrier preventing change. If the score does not change, you may have to use patience and persistence, and Troubleshoot. Just like with other Issues, beliefs can have Aspects that have to be changed.

On the other hand, you might wonder if beliefs can be changed from being not very true to being absolutely true. Yes, they can! First, you have to change the negative beliefs and painful memories that get in the way of the belief that you want. If you want to firmly believe "I am worthy of love and life," and the belief is hardly true for you, start by changing all the other negative beliefs and painful memories that seem related. This includes changing the belief "I am not worthy of love and life" to being not true. Then you simply set the Score for the wanted belief, say, 2 or 3, and hold the belief in your thoughts while tapping on the point behind your little finger and ring finger (see the 9-Gamut spot on page 30). Keep tapping and you can usually feel the truth of the belief gradually increase until it becomes totally true for you.

Remember, sometimes there are other beliefs or memories that have to be changed before the belief you're working on becomes absolutely true. If the process stalls at an 8 or a 9 or lower, and there is no change, ask yourself, "What stops this belief from becoming totally true?" Usually the answer will occur to you. You can use The Method to change the painful or inhibiting beliefs or memories that are stopping your desired belief from becoming totally true. After these barriers are changed, continue strengthening your desired belief.

It is important to make any beliefs that you desire empowering and attainable. Beliefs that involve your own feelings and emotions can be written very directly, like "I love and appreciate myself." But when constructing a positive belief that involves a response from your world, school, relationship or work, and so forth, you have to specify in the belief what you have to do to get the response from your world that gives you the feeling you want. This is the empowering aspect of the belief. So rather than setting your goal belief to "I am an A student," which may not be attainable, you would set it to be "When I study and apply myself, I can do my best in school." Setting empowering and attainable beliefs can be tricky. If you want to, discuss with a friend how to phrase your desired belief to make it empowering and attainable.

Compulsions and obsessive thoughts are based on beliefs and related internal dialogue that is motivated by Hurt. They can be much more complex than other memories and beliefs. Their repetitive nature in our thoughts interferes with the memory process. They are usually based on traumatic memories and beliefs that become preoccupying pastimes. Although they are difficult to change, it is still worth trying The Method. Often, by changing known traumatic memories and beliefs, you can end the compulsive behaviors and obsessive thoughts. If the sources of these behaviors are unknown to you, you can set up a schedule for using The Method to address the unconscious memories and the Hurt that causes them. Use the whole Method and a Phrase like "My fearful thoughts," or "My hand washing." Use a schedule and experiment with the frequency of The Method to see if the intensity or duration of the obsessive thoughts decrease. Do it for a month or so. You can also Troubleshoot. If all else fails, turn to Appendix V.

Some of you may like to have a daily Affirmation to reinforce who you want to become. Saying an Affirmation can gradually change how you feel about yourself and how you behave. But Affirmations are simply beliefs. Self-limiting behaviors, beliefs and traumatic memories can be barriers to experiencing your Affirmation. You can use The Method to clear away self-limiting behaviors, beliefs and memories that prevent you from being who you want to be. After clearing the barriers, you can strengthen the Affirmation you want later. By using The Method and the procedures described in this chapter, you may be able to speed up your rate of personal growth.

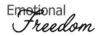

Chapter 14

Fixing the Need for a Fix: Getting Rid of Your Addiction(s)

If you have an addiction – whether it's drugs, alcohol, gambling or food – you know you do things you don't like that may disrupt your life. You know an addiction causes you pain and makes you miserable. Before you act on your addiction, whether it's lighting a cigarette or downing a drink, first you have an urge to engage in that addiction. The Method can heal the cause of those urges. When the cause is healed, the urge is gone. When the urge is gone, the addiction is gone. But it's not quite that simple.

There can be other traumatic memories or stress in your life that contribute to the addictive urges. Addictions can be a form of self-medication. Also, addictive urges appear to be triggered by situations where you have previously enjoyed the addiction. Sometimes the urge for an addiction can be unconscious. In this case, you can find yourself engaging in your addiction without consciously experiencing an urge. All the old traumas, stresses, remembered situations and unconscious motivations have to be resolved or changed to get rid of an addiction.

Using The Method gives you choice, because it gives you a way to neutralize your urge or craving whenever it occurs. Addictive urges are all based on Hurt. When you have an urge, you can eliminate it by using The Method. The Method gives you choices about how to respond to an addictive urge. With a sincere desire to beat an addiction, you can do The Method whenever you have an urge. If you take the drink or light up a cigarette, it's too late. The Method won't work. You have to do The Method while you have the urge, but before you engage in the addiction.

Since your addictive urges are stimulated by situations where you have done your addiction in the past, you can change the stimulating quality of these situations by using The Method on them. You can do this for any addiction. Here is a list of some situations pertaining to smoking: when I get up in the morning, at lunch, coffee break, problem solving, and so forth. Here are situations pertaining to food: at your mother's house, at the smorgasbord, pizza parlor, in front of the TV, and so forth. You can make a list of all the situations where you enjoy or do your addiction. Then, for each situation, create in your experience a strong addictive urge and do The Method. Lower the urge to 0. In this way you can also eliminate or reduce the urge before you are in the situation. Eating at a restaurant, for example, can cause intense cravings and overeating. Do The Method on the menu or the memory of the buffet to reduce the urge before you go to the restaurant. This will reduce your urge to eat excessively when you are actually in the restaurant (Callahan, 1991).

Our history of addiction often sabotages our intention to stop an addiction by providing us with barriers. This is the reason why the Affirmation is absolutely necessary for changing addictive urges. To make the Affirmation very effective, stimulate the urge or craving as strongly as you can. Use props like a cigarette pack, a candy wrapper, a smell, a dry drag on a cigarette, a beer can, a slice of cheesecake, a cookie or pepperoni, and so forth. Sometimes you have to get more intense, like taking the candy, unwrapping it, smelling it and taking small bites. Then, do The Method, including the Affirmation, with emphasis and conviction; cause some real soreness when rubbing the sore spot. Be careful not to bruise yourself. Use the Modified Affirmation often. Always do the Affirmation or Modified Affirmation. Do The Method until the Score of the craving goes to 0. Troubleshoot if necessary.

Because addictive urges can be motivated from your unconscious, you can never tell when they are going to hit. You suddenly experience yourself unconsciously walking into the store to buy a bottle of booze or some candy. You can gradually change this unconscious motivation by doing The Method on a schedule, say, every half hour. Over time, this behavior will no longer occur. When it does occur, do your best to eliminate the urge before you do the addiction. If you do the addiction, use the experience as feedback, and do The Method on the situation or start a repetition schedule. If you are already doing a schedule, make your schedule a little more intense by doing The Method more frequently. Try doing The Method before you leave home.

When you slip and do the addictive behavior, use the slip as feedback. Use The Method to change the situation or the thoughts that led you to do your addiction. Feel like a failure? Guilty? Other negative beliefs or self-destructive thoughts? Use The Method to change all those negative beliefs, self-destructive thoughts and feelings of failure and guilt. You don't need that Hurt. Strengthen the belief that your slip was a step toward changing the addiction by giving you a practical example of your addictive behavior. Strengthen the belief "I don't use drugs, smoke, or overeat, and so forth."

To eliminate addictive urges, try to follow these guidelines:

1. Address one addiction at a time. For example, change your addiction to drugs first, then alcohol, followed by cigarettes, and then food.

2. You may have to change your social activity or friends to stop your addiction.

3. You can increase your motivation to stop your addiction. Change any belief or situation that interferes with the belief "I want to stop my addiction." Use The Method to get this belief to be totally true for you (Callahan, 1991).

4. Do The Method on any traumatic memories that may be the basis for your addiction. If this is not possible, the repetition approach will probably work.

5. Always do The Method on the addictive urge by following a repetition schedule of 25 times per day until the urge no longer occurs. Fit the repetitions into your schedule or do them every half hour. Do not do The Method half-heartedly. Do it with enthusiasm and vigor. Use the Scheduling Form on page 45 to help you organize and do the schedule. It may take three to four days or longer to eliminate intense addictive urges.

6. Whenever you have an urge, set the Score for the urge to 10 and do The Method repeatedly until the urge goes away, that is, until the Score goes to 0.

7. If two applications of The Method result in no change in the Score, do the correction for a brain polarity (see page 40) before the Affirmation.

8. If the Score of the urge doesn't change, Troubleshoot. Frequently, chemicals or foods cause barriers to change, especially cigarettes and caffeine.

9. By using The Method, you can install the belief "I don't smoke" so it is true for you. Practice using this belief by doing The Method on the urge to smoke caused by the offer of a cigarette. You can do this by fantasizing a friend offering you a cigarette, and, while tapping on the 9-Gamut spot, saying to your friend in your fantasy, "Thank you, I don't smoke any more." Do this until the exchange feels really natural and true for you. Use this same approach to strengthen your defenses in any other situations where you think you will have a similar problem. This can be done with any addiction.

10. If you are changing your food addiction and your expected weight loss is moving too slowly for you, use The Method to change your feelings of impatience. Also use it to increase your patience for slow change (Callahan, 1991).

11. If you are trying to lose weight and have a long way to go, plan to lose 10 percent of your starting weight and then maintain that weight for three months. Then, lose 10 percent of your current weight and maintain that weight for three months. Continue in this way until you reach your goal weight. This strategy increases your ability to maintain your new weight by allowing your body, your eating habits and your self-image to adjust to the new weight (Aronne and Graver, 1998).

Withdrawal Symptoms

If you experience withdrawal symptoms, say, from cigarettes, coffee, alcohol or heroin, list all the symptoms and do the entire Method repeatedly for each symptom until the symptoms are gone. **Do not use any Shortcuts.** The emotional and physiological components underlying the withdrawal symptoms can be eliminated relatively easily, but the addictive urge or craving usually lasts for about three days.

Chapter 15

Reeducating Yourself:
If Your Symptoms Are Learned,
They Can Be Healed

Chronic illness sometimes causes painful memories. These are learned symptoms. During the most intense part of the course of a genuine illness (or trauma), memories of the symptoms, with varying degrees of Hurt, are often learned. Later, when the real physical cause of the pain and symptoms has been neutralized by medication or time, you might have chronic pain even though there is no medical reason for it. At this point, the pain is lingering like a bad odor. When this happens, the remembered pain causes the pain, because the physical reason for it has been healed. In short, you have chronic pain with no medical cause – remembered pain. When you apply The Method to this remembered pain, it usually dwindles to a Score of 0. It's gone.

If you have chronic symptoms and you have not seen a doctor about them, it is important to do so. Some symptoms may be an indication of a severe medical problem as yet undiagnosed. So if you have not seen a doctor before doing The Method on your symptoms, see your doctor, and rule out any systemic or structural problem.

Stress may be another cause for the intensity of your chronic symptoms. Stress causes tension in muscles. This tension, painful in its own right, can aggravate the physical damage, thereby increasing your Hurt. You can use The Method to eliminate your stress and, with luck, your chronic symptoms will be less painful.

Using The Method with learned symptoms is similar to what you have already learned to do. You do The Method on all the symptoms, one at a time. If the Score of the symptom decreases, you know you have changed the learned part of the symptom. To change it, you simply make a Phrase describing the symptom, set the Score, and do The Method on it. Begin without Shortcuts. Repeat The Method to bring the Score of the symptom down as low as you can. Remember, you are changing remembered Hurt, so if the symptom does not decrease to 0, there may be physical damage like a torn muscle, pulled ligament or a slipped disc, etc. However, it is always worth a try to change any chronic symptom just in case part of the symptom is remembered. If you have a barrier, Troubleshoot. If it still doesn't work, trying to change the Hurt of other symptoms may also be helpful. Be flexible and creative.

Here are the rules for approaching physical and chronic symptoms:

1. List the symptoms.

2. If you have not seen a doctor, see one before using The Method

3. Do The Method without Shortcuts. Start with the most severe symptom and work down, one by one, to the least severe symptom. Changing the big ones sometimes changes the small ones. This is opposite to the earlier approach for emotions, where you went from small to big.

4. With suspected physical damage, move your body or limb to clearly identify the extent of the Hurt. Do this when you assess the Score after doing The Method. Be sure that you take complete responsibility for yourself so that, if you move in some way to test an outcome, you won't Hurt yourself.

5. For a chronic disease with many symptoms, such as lupus, multiple sclerosis, carpal tunnel syndrome, and so forth, set up a schedule to do The Method 10 or more times a day. Use the Scheduling Form (see page 45) to schedule The Method. Expect to do the schedule for a month or more. Sometimes results are fast.

6. If you don't get results, try Troubleshooting.

7. Experiment by doing The Method more or fewer times per day. Explore how much you can change the intensity of the physical symptoms. See if there is a connection between the number of repetitions and the intensity of the Hurt. Determine the fewest replications of The Method it takes to keep the symptoms at a comfortable level.

8. For recurring symptoms like headaches, pain, upset stomach and constipation, and so forth, do The Method whenever you have the Hurt. This will probably change underlying memories that are causing the problems.

9. Sometimes diet and exercise habits have to be modified.

10. Attempt to eliminate all sources of stress in your life and daily activities. This may require changing your activities or your life style.

11. If your vocation is extremely stressful, consider looking for a less stressful vocation or place of employment.

Be patient and persistent. Sometimes the Hurt or symptoms shift from place to place in your body or experience. When one symptom changes, another shows up. It seems almost as if that by relaxing one symptom, another one is allowed to appear. Follow the changes. Do The Method on the symptoms as you become aware of them.

If The Method does not work immediately, turn to Troubleshooting, chapter ten. Always try doing The Method on a schedule. It is likely that you will find some relief. Remember, with physical damage in your body, the symptoms may never go to 0 or the symptoms may return. In either case, you can explore developing a program using The Method, as needed, to control the intensity of the symptoms.

Try The Method on anything and everything. It often works. It's easy, quick, and the results can be immediate. Also, when you use The Method to change a symptom, you can sometimes inadvertently change other underlying, emotional Issues.

Chapter 16

Working with the Inner You: Healing Negative Thoughts On Autopilot

The concept is called "Automatic Healing." I know it sounds unusual, but it is the direction in which science and my clinical practice have been moving for quite some time. I've thought quite a bit about whether to include this information, and I've concluded that those people who accept the ideas in this chapter will truly enjoy putting the idea of automatic healing into practice. As strange as it sounds, these ideas offer two major benefits: They will let you make your own healing process automatic, and you will be able to use that process on demand. All you have to do is read. These ideas are embedded in statements that will teach your Innerself how to heal.

The statements offered below for the Innerself are based, in part, on ideas used in hypnosis; but it is not hypnosis. When you talk to your Innerself in the course of reading a statement, you can bet that you are not in a hypnotic trance. A caveat is warranted, however. Readers with religious beliefs against, or considerations about, doing anything that is connected to the Innerself or hypnosis can skip this chapter. You can use The Method very effectively without the content of this chapter.

Therapists and others have been working with the Innerself for years. This is a common practice of hypnotherapists and other treatment approaches based in part on hypnosis. The following strategy is the culmination of my work in using The Method (Craig and Fowlie, 1995), Thought Field Therapy™ (Callahan, 1985, 1991, 1993) and the Tapas Acupressure Technique (Fleming, 1998). Some of it is based on recent scientific findings, and other parts of it are based on various treatment methodologies and clinical experience. Regardless, I believe that it is easy to learn and will work for many people.

In this chapter, you will be given a statement that will alert your Innerself that it can use The Method as an internal healing process. Then, with this revelation, the Innerself can use The Method to remove barriers to our natural healing processes. Further statements will be offered that will reveal that heart energy and cellular sensitivity to people who love and care for you can be used to facilitate the healing process. With this, the Innerself will be asked to automatically heal all negative beliefs, memories and experience that enter into your conscious and unconscious activity. Then you will have examples of using the Innerself to change specific negative emotions, beliefs and memories and to strengthen positive beliefs.

Teaching the Innerself

We all have insights, gut feelings, and other experiences that surprise us. We attribute the origin of some of these experiences to our subconscious or Innerself. Some people believe that each of us has an Innerself that has access to all our experience, from birth or even conception, to now. This is the part of us that hypnotherapists access when the main personality is put to sleep. The joke is that the Innerself never sleeps and is always aware of what is going on. So it is possible to talk to it while you are watching TV, riding your bicycle or brushing your teeth. After you read the following paragraph, your Innerself will have an *aha* experience from learning that it is possible for him/her to do The Method as an internal healing process to change Issues. The following statement is intended to alert the Innerself that learning an internal healing process is possible. Read the statement out loud.

> I want my Innerself to review the information on The Method and on Troubleshooting. Know that by carefully observing The Method as I do it, you can learn how to mimic the technique to assist me. With the instructions you'll receive, you will also be able to do the change process without any prompting from me or anyone else.

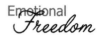

Remove the Barriers to Natural Healing

We have all heard stories of people who have experienced miracle cures from cancer and other terminal illnesses. These are interpreted to be examples of our body's mobilizing to heal itself using its own natural healing processes. This happened because some of these survivors worked very hard to remove barriers to get their natural healing processes to work. Let's look at it from another direction. It is commonly known that persons who have had severe trauma can sometime heal cuts and injuries at an incredible pace (Braun, 1983). How can this happen? Here is how I think it happens.

With severe trauma, an aspect of our personality can be separated from the main personality via a massive survival response. During a severe trauma, the brain generates behavior independent of our main personality. The intensity of this survival activity pushes the main personality to sleep, an inactive state in the brain. This survival activity becomes an aspect or part of our personality. These parts, separated from the main personality by amnesia, have not learned that the body cannot heal itself. Therefore, when a trauma-based part is active, the body may operate using the natural processes of healing without the learned barriers that otherwise slow down or block the healing process when the main personality is active. These persons with a history of severe trauma sometimes heal physical problems with surprising speed.

Barriers to natural healing are, in a sense, similar to the barriers that stop The Method from working. Sometimes we have to use an Affirmation to get The Method to work. The use of the Affirmation is a way to clear our experience so the memory process can work. There are other, more subtle barriers that prevent your brain and body from using its natural healing processes. The subtle barriers have to do with the beliefs and memories that support the belief that we cannot heal or change our own physical problems or Issues. That's why we go to physicians, therapists and alternative healing disciplines. These subtle barriers block the full use of our natural healing processes. The barriers are the beliefs and memories we have learned from parents, ourselves, our reading, the medical industry and others who have given us external fixes for aches, pains, illnesses and disease. It is possible for your Innerself to heal these barriers using The Method. After these barriers are healed, the natural healing processes will be more likely to work when you do The Method and as well as when the subconscious engages in the use of The Method to heal something.

Here is a task that may change all those self-limiting beliefs and memories that interfere with fully using your natural healing processes when you use The Method or simply want to change something. The following statement will assign a task to the Innerself that facilitates the natural healing process specifically by using The Method to eliminate all beliefs and memories that present subtle barriers to the belief that you can heal yourself. Read the following statement out loud.

> Innerself, will you go back as far as you have to and change all beliefs and memories from then until now that interfere with my spontaneous use of my natural healing processes. After you finish that, please strengthen the belief that "I am capable of healing all learned physical and mental Issues with natural healing processes."

Bringing the Heart Field to the Healing Process

Recent research has shown that the heart has a much greater influence on our experience and behavior than previously believed. Pearsall(1998) describes how heart transplant recipients often have experiences and show behaviors that are similar to the heart donor. He goes on to suggest that the heart is communicating with the brain and all cells in the body via a subtle electromagnetic field. Similarly, Bruce Lipton(1995, 1998) has discussed how individual cells are sensitive to electromagnetic fields. He goes on to say that our cells are constantly bathed in the electromagnetic fields generated by the neural activity of the brain and other organs of the body. Since the heart is known to put out the most intense field in the body, and the cells in the brain and body respond to it, it may be that the heart field can participate in the change process. My recent clinical findings support this hypothesis.

Let's look at electromagnetic field impact from another direction. During a trauma, the brain uses memories of experience and behavior to try to escape. Because cells are sensitive to electromagnetic fields, sometimes negative fields of perpetrators or others are learned by the brain during its highly mobilized state in a trauma. The "field learnings" might be information that is possibly useful in escaping the trauma. These field learnings become connected to traumatic memories, behaviors, or beliefs. When present, negative field learnings both interfere with change and support dysfunction by evoking motivating emotions for the behavior, belief or memory. See Kraft (1993) for an interesting discussion of other phenomena.

The following statement requests the Innerself to use the heart field in the change processes and instructs the Innerself to invite any of the negative field learnings to be changed by using the power of the heart field. Also, if you wish, include spiritual requests in the following statements where appropriate. Don't forget to read out loud.

> Innerself, use that internal response that elicits the most intense heart field and use the heart field in all change processes. If ever there are any negative field learnings serving as a barrier, combine these fields with the strongest field and elicit an intense heart field to change the quality of the negative field learnings.

Awakening Your Sensitivity to Field Stimulation

Although controversial, Therapeutic Touch is taught to nurses in many medical schools and worldwide in over 75 countries. It has been shown to have a marked impact on hospitalized patients (Krieger, 1993). It is used widely in many applications. This practice, in my opinion, is similar to techniques that were popular in the 19th century before analgesics were discovered. Without elaborating, the healing power of stroking close to the body appears to be well documented, though seldom used or accepted in clinical psychology. It involves the healing power of the heart field – love and compassion, and other resources that the practitioner can give and use with a person who has a physical illness or pain. The repeated stroking of the arm apparently sensitizes both bodies to the field generated by the practitioner and the patient. Some aspect of this experience seems to facilitate reduction in pain or an increased rate of healing. By demonstrating this field connection between two people to your Innerself, the Innerself can mimic the cellular sensitivity throughout your body that will increase the effectiveness of your healing processes.

Another consequence of experiencing the field connection is that the experience may awaken your awareness of the connection to the heart field of others who care for you (Pearsall, 1998). Both may be helpful in self-healing. Krieger (1993) has noted that the Therapeutic Touch is effective for relaxation, pain reduction, stimulating healing processes and changing the cause and intensity of symptoms. You have learned that you can use The Method on all these Issues, so we are adding the Therapeutic Touch experience for the Innerself who can later mimic the experience in the healing process.

The following task is designed to teach your Innerself to experience the effects of Therapeutic Touch so that it can use the learnings to facilitate inner healing whether as a local process or as a process that involves others. This requires asking a friend to help you. It's the impact of your friend's heart field that can teach you the cell response or brain response that may be useful in increasing the effectiveness of your internal healing processes. Here's how to do it.

Find a trusted friend. While your friend focuses on his or her love for you or someone he or she particularly loves, at the same time have them slowly stroke your arm about 1 to 2 inches above the surface. Start at the shoulder and move slowly down your arm and off your fingertips in about 4 to 5 seconds. Have the person stroke your arm repeatedly in this way until you feel a sensation in your arm caused by the stroking. When you feel it, read the following statement out loud:

> Innerself, feel the effect of the field influence on my arm and learn to use all aspects of this experience throughout our body, whenever needed, to help with my internal healing processes.

Automatically Change Negative Beliefs and Memories

The Innerself is always awake. It can constantly monitor our activity and spontaneously change all negative beliefs, experiences and memories that occur in our conscious or unconscious experience. It can also strengthen positive beliefs that will bring you more satisfaction. In this way, we can gradually change to have a more satisfying life. Read this statement out loud.

> Innerself, remove all negativity from any beliefs, experiences or memories that occur to me, consciously or unconsciously, in the normal course of life. Strengthen related positive, self-empowering beliefs. If anger is involved, please heal the anger and strengthen an experience of heartfelt forgiveness.

Change Specific Negative Emotions, Beliefs or Memories

Negative emotions, beliefs, experiences and memories can also be changed by using your Innerself. You simply ask your Innerself to change or eliminate the emotions connected to the Issue. You can probably change most or all Issues by asking your Innerself. Here are a couple of examples:

1. You were always told you were pretty when you grew up, but your sister was the beauty queen in the family. You have the belief that you are unattractive. Change this by saying the following statement to yourself:

Innerself, please weaken the belief "I am unattractive."

Assess the Score of the truth and see if you can feel the truth of the belief gradually decrease. You can also strengthen positive beliefs.

2. You arrived home and found that your dog ripped up your down pillow, leaving feathers all over the house. You feel like abusing the dog. Go into another room without the dog, close the door and say the following to your Innerself:

Innerself, please reduce my anger with my dog.

Assess the Score of your anger. See if you can feel the anger with your dog gradually decline.

Strengthening Desired, Positive Beliefs

In a similar way, the Innerself can strengthen beliefs that we want to experience more fully. Rather than continuously tapping on the 9-Gamut spot, you simply ask your Innerself to strengthen the belief. Of course, you must be aware of two things. First, the belief has to be self-empowering (see page 54) and, second, there may be some barriers to strengthening the belief, so before strengthening a belief, ask your Innerself to remove any negative beliefs and memories that stand in the way of strengthening the belief. Here is an example of strengthening a belief:

Innerself, please strengthen the belief "I am worthy of love and worthy of life."

When you ask the Innerself to strengthen a belief, see if you can feel the truth of the belief gradually increase.

No Guarantee

There is no guarantee that these statements or this Innerself healing process will work for you. You may not be able to activate an ongoing change process. We are all different. There can be unknown parts of our personality that feel suspicious of change itself, or parts that have so much pain that they are afraid to allow any change fearing that the change process could cause a destructive flood of emotions or behavior. These parts can stop the change process. But your Innerself can also know that parts with enormous pain or a self-damaging tendency can be changed very, very slowly. This is done by changing, in slow steps, only a small amount of the pain of the trauma that will be less than the pain just noticeable by the person. Other barriers may need Troubleshooting. Nevertheless, it is worth trying these statements again, to see if you can obtain a natural healing process working spontaneously. The statements are listed in Appendix III for your convenience. **But**, on the other hand, your Innerself has probably already felt the *aha.*

As a point of interest, sometimes when an internal healing process is going on you can feel sensations in your brain or scalp. I interpret these experiences as the rapid change of memory associations.

Chapter 17

The Last Few Comments

There you have it. Now you can use The Method to help you remove Hurt from Issues and blast through many, if not all, of your life's barricades. That means breaking out of the inhibiting beliefs, painful memories and traumas that are holding you back. You can master your addictions and point your life in whatever direction you choose. Sometimes you'll even be able to relieve physical and medical afflictions if part of the symptoms is learned. That is the power of The Method, a power you can use for the rest of your life.

Now is the time to get started. List your Issues, develop the Aspects, and order the Issues and Aspects from least Hurtful to most Hurtful (see page 17). Remember, a series of small Issues successfully changed will build your confidence in The Method. Select a minor Issue that is not connected to trauma but has the largest hurt. Don't forget to use common sense. You will know if it is a biggie. Change the minor Issue with The Method. Notice the results.

Frequently, results happen so fast that people think up other reasons to explain the change, like "I was simply distracted" or "It wasn't anything anyway" (Callahan, 1991). You may have these thoughts, but continue to work through your Issues. The Method will work if you use the contents of this book with patience and persistence.

Most problems usually are not difficult to change. But if you run into any difficulties and have exhausted your patience with Troubleshooting, you can turn to Appendix V for other options. It may be possible to provide you with a referral to a therapist in your area familiar with this approach. The strategies for getting additional help are given in Appendix V.

If you have any thoughts about this book, please fill in the feedback form on page 93. I would also like to hear about your successful and unsuccessful outcomes with Issues or the healing process. Let me know about other Issues that are not listed.

Disclaimer

Don't forget to see a doctor if you have an acute pain or illness or if you have been having any ongoing pain or sensation. It is very important to take care of yourself, and seeing a doctor regularly or as needed.

Appendix I

Issues, Aspects, and Phrases

Emotion Issues

Issue	Aspect	Phrase
Generic	I have this problem.	This problem
Anger	I have this anger.	This anger
Anorexia	I am afraid of looking fat.	Fear of looking fat
	I am afraid of getting fat.	Fear of getting fat
	I have a fear of eating food.	This fear of eating
	I have a fear of eating some foods.	This fear
	Note: Always use the Affirmation.	
Anxiety	I have this anxiety.	This anxiety
	I have this terror.	This terror
Ashamed	I always feel ashamed.	Feeling ashamed
Auto accident	(see Motor vehicle accident)	
Back injury	(see Pain)	
Body embarrassment	My body embarrasses me.	My embarrassment
	This scar upsets me.	This upset
	(Blemish, pimple, etc.)	
Body shame	I am ashamed of my body.	My shame
Boredom	I have this boredom.	This boredom
Bulimia	(see Anorexia)	
Chronic anxiety	I always feel anxious.	Anxious feelings
Claustrophobia	I feel trapped.	Fear of being trapped
	I am afraid to go outside.	Fear of going out
Claustrophobia in car	I am afraid to be in the car.	Fear in car
	I am afraid when the car is running.	My fear
	I am afraid when the car is moving.	Moving car
	I am terrified that we will crash.	Auto crash
	I am afraid that I can't get out.	Being trapped
	I am afraid of heavy traffic.	Fear of traffic
Death of loved one	I can't talk about the death of my	My sadness
	I feel sad about the death of my	My sadness

Issue	Aspect	Phrase
Depression	I am depressed.	This depression
	I am depressed that	This depression
	I am angry that	This anger
	I feel hopeless	Hopeless feelings
	(Worthless, other symptoms)	
Emotions, unidentified	I have these emotions.	These emotions
Fear of crowds	I am afraid of crowds.	Fear of crowds
	I am afraid to go into restaurants.	Fear of restaurants
	I have to have my back to the wall.	This fear
	I have to spot the exits.	This fear
	I look for potential danger in crowds.	Fear of danger
	I am intensely aware of potential harm.	Fear of getting hurt
	I feel anxious in crowded places.	This anxiety
	I feel paranoid.	My paranoia
	I feel like a target in crowds.	My fear
Fear of dentists	I am afraid of experiencing pain.	Fear of pain
	Dental office smell frightens me.	Dentist smell
	I am afraid of the grinding.	Fear of grinding
	Getting my teeth cleaned is scary.	Cleaning fear
Fear of elevators	I am afraid of elevators.	Fear of elevators
	I am afraid of closed places.	Fear of closed places
Fear of flying	I am afraid of flying.	Fear of flying
	I am afraid of dying.	Fear of dying
	I am afraid of crashing.	Fear of crashing
	I am afraid of landing.	Fear of landing
	I am afraid of taking off.	Fear of taking off
	I am afraid of the wings falling off.	This fear
	I am claustrophobic.	Being trapped
Fear of the future	I am afraid of what's going to happen.	Fear of future
	I am afraid of the future of the planet.	My planet fears
Fear of needles	I'm afraid of needles.	Fear of needles
Fear of rats	I am afraid of the tail.	Fear of the tail
	I am afraid I'll get bitten.	Fear of rat bite
	I feel anxious with rats and mice.	My anxiety
	I have this challenge with rats.	Fear of rats
Fear of riding in cars	I am anxious when I get into the car.	Anxiety in car
	I am anxious when car is turned on.	My anxiety
	I am anxious when it is in traffic.	Anxiety in traffic
	I am afraid I will get in a crash.	Fear of crash
	I am afraid I can't get out.	Fear of being trapped
Fear of snakes	I am afraid of getting bitten.	Fear getting bitten
	I am afraid it will crawl on me.	This fear
	I am afraid of it will crawl on my face.	This fear
	I had a trauma(s) with a snake.	Fear of snakes

Issue	Aspect	Phrase
Fear of water	I am afraid of water.	Fear of water
	I am afraid I am going to die.	Fear of dying
	I am afraid I'll drown.	Fear of drowning
	I am afraid a fish will bite me.	Fear of fish
	I am afraid to dunk my head.	Dunking my head
	I am afraid when I can't see the bottom.	My fear
	I am afraid when water is over my chin.	Water over chin
	When my mouth goes under water, I am afraid I'll need air.	This fear
Global planetary fear	(see Fear of the future.)	
Grief	I have deep sadness about his/her death.	My sadness
	I am afraid to talk about his/her death.	My fear
	I feel anger now.	My anger
Guilt	I feel guilty that I . . . (specify)	My guilt
	I feel guilty that I hit my	My guilt
	I have this terrible memory and extreme guilt.	This memory
Headache	I have anxiety headaches.	Anxiety headache
	I have a headache.	This headache
	I have a migraine headache.	Migraine
	Note: Try on any headache.	
Hiccups	I have these hiccups.	Hiccups
Being over water	I am afraid of being over water.	Fear of water
	I am afraid of snakes in the water.	Snakes in water
	I am afraid of dark water.	Fear of dark water
	I am afraid when I am alone over water.	Alone over water
Height phobia	I am afraid of heights.	Fear of height
	I am afraid I am going to fall.	Fear of falling
	I have anxiety that I am going to fall.	Falling anxiety
	I am afraid I'll hurt myself if I fall.	Fear of injury
	When I am on a ladder, I am afraid.	Fear of height
Inadequacy feelings	I feel inadequate.	These feelings
	I am afraid of failure.	Fear of failure
	I am afraid of success.	Fear of success
Insomnia	I can't go to sleep.	Can't sleep
	I wake up at 4 a.m.	Wake up early
	I have insomnia.	Insomnia
Intrusive memory	I have an intrusive memory.	This memory
	My intrusive memories freak me out.	My fear

Note: Change one memory at a time.
Tell the story about the memory and do
The Method on any Hurt that is experienced.
Repeat until there is no remaining Hurt.

Issue	Aspect	Phrase
Love pain	I am afraid to get into a relationship.	Fear of relationship
	I am afraid she will say no.	Fear of rejection
	I am anxious when I am with her.	My anxiety
	I am afraid that she will drop me.	Fear of rejection
Motor vehicle accident	I felt anxious that something was wrong.	My anxiety
	I was upset and frightened after the accident.	These feelings
	I was terrified when I hit.	Terror
	I was afraid in the ambulance.	That fear
	I was terrified when the gas was dripping on my chest.	That terror
Pain	I have neck pain.	Neck pain
	I have lower back pain.	Back pain
	I have joint pains.	Joint pain
	I have rib pain.	Rib pain
	I have corn pains.	Corn pain
	I have hip pain.	Hip pain
	I have pains in my knees.	Knee pain
	I have a pain in my shoulder.	Shoulder pain
	(Later)	Remaining pain
	I have this tightness.	This tightness
Panic attack	I have this panic.	This panic
Phobias	(see Fear of)	
Posttraumatic stress	I have intrusive memories.	These memories
	I have a "symptom."	This "symptom"
	I feel guilty that I	This guilt
	Note: See also Anxiety, Headache, Guilt, Grief and Traumatic memory.	
Public speaking	I am afraid to speak in groups.	Fear of groups
	I am anxious when I talk to groups.	My anxiety
Sadness	I always feel sad.	My sadness
Self-image	(see Body-image, Inadequacy)	
Sexual abuse	(see Posttraumatic stress, Self-image, etc.)	
Social withdrawal	I feel anxious with people.	Anxiety with people
	I feel sadness.	My sadness
	I feel anger.	My anger
	I feel deep sadness.	My deep sadness
	Note: Change the most intense sad experience and any other memory that makes you sad or anxious.	

Issue	Aspect	Phrase
Spiders	I am afraid of spiders.	Fear of spiders
	I am afraid of a moving spider.	Moving spider
Sports, golf	I have tension when I swing my club.	This tension
	I feel anxious when I hear noise.	Hearing noise
	I am afraid to succeed.	Fear of success
Stress	(see Anxiety)	
Swallowing	I have fear of swallowing food.	Fear of swallowing
Throat discomfort	I have a painful throat.	This painful throat
Traumatic memory	I have intrusive memories.	These memories
	I feel terror when I remember	This terror
	I failed when I	My failure
	I was in terror when I felt something going wrong.	My terror
	I am fearful of my memory.	My fear
	Note: Play memory through like a movie to search for Hurt.	
War memory	(see Traumatic memory)	
Withdrawal, social	I feel anxious with people.	This anxiety
	I feel sadness.	My sadness
	I feel anger.	My anger
	I feel deep sadness.	My deep sadness

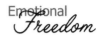

Addictions

In general, list all the situations where you have done your addiction. Do The Method on the addictive urge experienced in each situation until you can think of all the situations without creating an addictive urge. As more situations are remembered or urges experienced, eliminate the urge by doing The Method.

Issue	Aspect	Phrase
Alcoholism	I crave drinking beer.	Craving
	I want a drink when I get up.	Getting up
	I like to sneak drinks at work.	Sneaking drinks
	I like to drink with my friends.	With my friends
Candy	I want to eat this candy.	This candy
Chocolate	I constantly crave chocolate.	Craving chocolate
	I have a challenge with chocolate.	Chocolate challange
	I crave the chocolate when I see it.	Chocolate
	I crave the candy when I unwrap it.	Unwrapping the candy
	I crave it when I smell it.	This smell of candy
	I crave it when I taste it.	This taste of candy
Coffee addiction	I want a cup of coffee.	Want coffee
Drug addiction	I have an urge to smoke marijuana.	Urge to smoke

Remember: List all the situations where you used drugs. For each situation, generate an urge for the drug and eliminate the urge with The Method. Use The Method whenever an urge arises.

Smoking	I crave that cigarette.	Crave that cigarette
	(Later)	Remaining craving
Soft drinks	I crave a "soft drink."	Crave a "soft drink"
Withdrawal symptoms	I have this symptom.	This symptom
(Identify	I have the sweats.	The sweats
all symptoms)	I have the shakes.	This shaking

Note: With some medical Issues, The Method should be done in a doctor's presence.

Chronic Illnesses
and Physical Problems

Issue	Aspect	Phrase
Allergies	I have this allergy.	This allergy
	I have an allergy to milk.	Milk allergy
Asthma	I have asthma.	Asthma
Back injury	(see Pain)	
Breathing problem	I have a breathing problem.	Breathing problem
Burning eyes	I have burning eyes.	My burning eyes
Cancer symptoms	(Do The Method on each symptom.)	This "symptom"
Constipation	I am constantly constipated.	My constipation
Dyslexia	I feel anxious when I read.	Reading anxiety
	I feel anxious when I read aloud.	My reading aloud
	I feel anxious when I spell.	My spelling anxiety
Fingernail biting	I bite my fingernails.	My nail-biting
Headache	I have anxiety headaches.	Anxiety headache
	I have a headache.	This headache
	I have a migraine headache.	This migraine
Hiccups	I have these hiccups.	These hiccups
Insomnia	I can't go to sleep.	Can't sleep
	I wake up at 4 a.m.	My waking early
	I have insomnia.	My insomnia
Irritable bowel syndrome	I have irritable bowel syndrome.	This syndrome
Lupus	I have lupus disease.	My lupus disease
	I have a stomach ache.	My stomach ache
	I feel nauseated.	This nausea
	I have a neck ache.	This neck ache

Note: List symptoms and do The Method on all symptoms.

Issue	Aspect	Phrase
Multiple sclerosis	(see Lupus)	
Needles	I'm afraid of needles.	Fear of needles
Numbness in fingers	I have numb fingers.	My numb fingers

Issue	Aspect	Phrase
Pain	I have this neck pain.	My neck pain
	I have lower back pain.	My back pain
	I have joint pains.	My joint pain
	I have corn pains.	My corn pain
	I have hip pain.	My hip pain
	I have pains in my knees.	My knee pain
	I have a pain in my shoulder.	My shoulder pain
	(Later)	Remaining pain

Note: Sometimes when one pain is healed, the pain reduction generalizes to other pain sites. The pain does not go to 0 if there is a mechanical problem.

Issue	Aspect	Phrase
Pre-Menstural Syndrome	I have terrible PMS.	PMS symptoms
Sinus related problem	I have postnasal drip.	Postnasal drip
Swallowing	Fear of swallowing food.	My fear of swallowing
Throat discomfort	I have this throat feeling.	My throat feeling
Ulcerative colitis	I have ulcerative colitis.	My ulcerative colitis

Cautions:

1. With some medical Issues, The Method should be done in a doctor's presence.

2. If you move in some way to test an outcome of The Method, take complete responsibility for your well-being by being careful to not hurt yourself.

Appendix II

Reminders

It is all right to photocopy this page and place these handy cards in your wallet or purse.

Remember the order:

Affirmation
Sequence
9-Gamut
Sequence

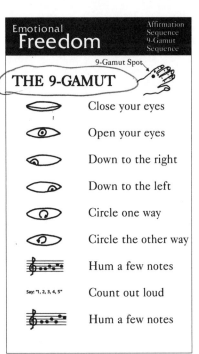

Appendix III

Innerself Healing

After you use The Method a number of times, these are the statements you can read to see if you can successfully internalize The Method. Don't forget to include spiritual requests if it is appropriate for you to do so. Reread these statements out loud.

Teaching the Innerself

I want my Innerself to review the information on The Method and on Troubleshooting. Know that by carefully observing The Method as I do it, you can learn how to mimic the technique and assist me. With the instructions you'll receive, you will also be able to do the change process without any prompting from me or anyone else.

Reread the chapter ten on Troubleshooting at this time (see page 38).

Remove Barriers to Natural Healing

Innerself, will you go back as far as you have to and change all beliefs and memories from then until now that interfere with the spontaneous use of my natural healing processes. After you finish that, please strengthen the belief "I am capable of healing all learned physical and mental Issues with natural healing processes."

Bringing the Heart Field to the Healing Process

Innerself, use that internal response that elicits the most intense heart field and use the heart field in all change processes. If ever there are any negative field learnings serving as a barrier, combine these fields with the strongest field and elicit the intense heart field to change the quality of the field learning.

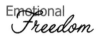

Awakening Your Sensitivity to Field Stimulation

Have a friend stroke your arms as described on page 69, feel the field stimulation and read the following statement:

> Innerself, feel the effect of the field influence on my arm and learn to use all aspects of this experience throughout our body, whenever needed, to help with my internal healing processes.

Automatically Change Negative Beliefs and Memories

> Innerself, remove all negativity from any beliefs, experiences or memories that occur to me, consciously or unconsciously, in the normal course of life. Strengthen related positive, self-empowering beliefs. If anger is involved, please heal the anger and strengthen an experience of heartfelt forgiveness.

Experiment with the Innerself to see if you can heal emotions, negative beliefs and memories by simply asking the Innerself to do it. Also, try to strengthen beliefs that you want to be totally true for you. Remember about the self-empowering Issue (see page 54) and that sometimes you have to change negative beliefs or memories before you can strengthen the truth of a positive belief.

Do you remember when you changed your history to remove the barriers that prevented you from believing that you could heal yourself? You can also give the same change history request to your Innerself to change the effects of any negative learned pattern that you have, such as that caused by a painful childhood experience, school experience, job experience or relationship, and so forth. You can ask your Innerself to change the effects of that negative experience from when it happened to now. If appropriate for you, you can ask your Innerself to create a feeling of forgiveness for the person that caused a negative experience.

Appendix IV

References

Aronne, L. J. & Graver, F. (1995). Weigh Less, Live Longer. New York: Wiley.

Braun, G. B. (1983). Psychophysiologic Phenomena in Multiple Personality and Hypnosis. American J. of Hypnosis, 26, 124-137.

Callahan, R. J. (1981). Psychological Reversal. Collected Papers of the International College of Applied Kinesiology, Winter, 79-96.

Callahan, R. J. (1985). Five Minute Phobia Cure. Wilmington, DE: Enterprise.

Callahan, R. J. (1991). Why Do I Eat When I Am Not Hungry? New York: Avon Books.

Callahan, R. J. (1993). Diagnostic training in Thought Field Therapy, Indian Wells, California.

Callahan, R. J. (2001). Tapping the Healer Within: Using Thought Field Therapy to Instantly Conquer Your Fears, Anxieties, and Emotional Distress. Chicago, IL: Contemporary Books.

Craig, G. H. & Fowlie, A. (1995). Emotional Freedom Techniques: The Manual. Sea Ranch, CA: Author.

Durlacher, J. V. (1995). Freedom From Fear Forever. Tempe, AZ: Van Ness Publishing.

Figley, C. R. (1995). Posted on traumatic-stress@freud.apa.org. 11-95 by Charles R. Figley, Ph. D., Florida State University, Tallahassee, FL.

Figley, C. and Carbonell, J. (1995-1997). <u>Study of the Active
Ingredients of PTSD Cures.</u> At a conference sponsored by
the Psychological Stress Research Program and Clinical
Laboratory. Florida State University, Tallahassee, FL.

Fleming, T. (1998). <u>You Can Heal Now: The Tapas Acupressure
Technique (TAT).</u> TAT International, Redondo Beach,
CA: Author.

Flint, G. A. (In Press). A Chaos Model of the Brain Applied to
EMDR. In A. Cooms (Ed.), <u>Mind in Time.</u> Cresskill, NJ:
Hampton Press.

Flint, G. A. (1994, June). <u>Toward a Chaos Model of Memory: A
Model Based Upon Clinical Methodology.</u> Paper presented
at the 1994 Annual Conference of the Society for Chaos
Theory in Psychology and the Life Sciences, Baltimore,
MD.

Flint, G. A. (1997, June). <u>A Learning Model of the Personality:
From Explanation to Intervention.</u> Workshop presented at
the 5th International Congress on the Disorders of
Personality, Vancouver, BC, Canada.

Goodheart, G. J., Jr. (1964-1978). <u>Applied Kinesiology: Workshop
Method Manual.</u> Ed. 1-14. Privately Published.

Kraft, C. H. (1993). <u>Deep Wounds, Deep Healing.</u> Ann Arbor, MI:
Servant Publications.

Krieger, D. (1993). <u>Accepting Your Power to Heal: The Personal
Practice of Therapeutic Touch.</u> Santa Fe, NM: Bear &
Company.

Lipton, B. (1995). <u>The Invisible Biology.</u> A workshop presented at
the Frontiers of Hypnosis conference sponsored by the
Canadian Society of Clinical Hypnosis – Alberta Division,
Banff, AB, Canada.

Lipton, B. (1998, November). <u>How Beliefs Become Heredity: An Introduction to Cellular Psychology.</u> Workshop given at the 15th international conference of the International Society for the Study of Dissociation, Seattle, WA.

Pearsall, P. (1998). <u>The Heart's Code.</u> New York: Broadway Books.

Walther, D. S. (1981). <u>Applied Kinesiology: Basic Procedures and Muscle Testing. Vol 1.</u> Pueblo, CO: SDC Systems.

Walther, D. S. (1988). <u>Applied Kinesiology: Synopsis.</u> Pueblo, CO: SDC Systems.

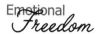

Appendix V

Resources

If you have difficulties, questions or need assistance in finding a therapist, contact Gary Craig's web site or myself.

Gary Craig's web site:
> To obtain training, treatment information or help in locating a therapist, go to this web site:
> Web site: http://www.emofree.com

Garry A. Flint:
> Telephone: (250) 558-5077 Fax: (250) 558-5044
> E-Mail: gaflint@emotional-freedom.com
> Web site: http://www.emotional-freedom.com

How to find a good therapist:

✓ Contact Gary Craig's web site to see if there is a trained therapist in your area.

✓ Call a local, state or province professional association and ask if they can give you a name of a therapist who is trained in either Thought Field Therapy™ or Emotional Freedom Techniques.

✓ Call local counselors, social workers, or psychologists and ask if they know the name of a licensed or registered therapist trained in Thought Field Therapy™ or Emotional Freedom Techniques. If they don't know of one, ask if they know of someone who might know.

✓ Call the local woman's shelter or safe house and ask if they can recommend a therapist who is trained in Thought Field Therapy™ or Emotional Freedom Techniques. If you have some names of some therapists, ask if they think these therapists are good.

✓ If the above fails, repeat your calls and ask if they know of a Certified Trauma Specialist or a good therapist trained in EMDR. Frequently these therapists are well trained and good at changing Hurt.

Call the appropriate licensing board to see if the therapist is currently licensed and if any disciplinary actions have been filed against him or her.

If you are interested in finding out more about this type of therapy and other effective therapies, go to your computer or a friend's computer and visit the following web sites:

http://tftrx.com (Thought Field Therapy)

http://www.emofree.com (Emotional Freedom Techniques)

http://www.energypsych.com (Energy Diagnostic and Treatment Methods)

Other therapies that are also powerful can be reviewed at the following web sites:

http://www.tat-intl.com (Tapas Acupressure Techniques)

http://www.emdr.com (Eye Movement Desensitization and Reprocessing)

For trauma in general, go to:

http://www.trauma-pages.com (An award winning web site)

Appendix VI

Give Feedback

I would like your feedback. Please cut out and fax or mail the following form to me so I can assess the effectiveness of this book in teaching The Method. If you have any suggestions about how to improve the clarity of the book, please feel free to photocopy pages of the book, mark them up, and return them to me.

I would like you to list all the Issues for which you found The Method effective. Also list the Issues for which you could not make The Method work. I also would like to know if you found the chapter on Innerself healing useful.

Any and all comments are welcome. Feel free to use additional pages.

Thank you in advance.

Garry A. Flint, Ph.D.

Mail or fax to:

Garry A. Flint, Ph.D.
#5 - 2906 32nd Street
Vernon, BC, Canada V1T 5M1
Fax: (250) 558-5044

Place of Purchase: _____

Today's Date: _____

The Method worked for me. __ Yes __ No

Here is a list of Issues I changed to a comfortable score:

_____

_____

_____

Here is a list of Issues I was unable to change:

_____

_____

_____

Did you share this book with others? __ Yes __ No

Did the Innerself healer work for you? __ Yes __ No

Please use a separate sheet to make any additional comments.

Thank you for giving me this feedback.

Garry A. Flint, Ph.D.

Index

D

E

F

G

H

I

About the Author

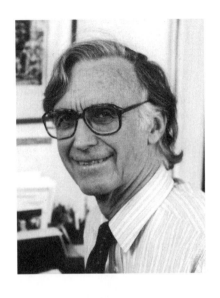

Garry A. Flint was educated at Indiana University and, in 1968, received a doctoral degree in experimental psychology specializing in learning. He ended up in Ukiah, California, where, after working with abused teens for six years, he became a staff psychologist at the county mental health outpatient clinic. He continued to work with abused children and adults. Here, he began to search for treatment techniques that worked faster than Behavior Modification. He obtained extensive training in hypnosis and Neurolinguistic Programming. Later, he was the program manager of a psychiatric health facility where he was able to work with severely disturbed persons. In 1987 he started a private practice. In 1990 he was further trained in Eye Movement Desensitization and Reprocessing (EMDR). Before moving to Canada in 1994, he took the diagnostic training for Thought Field Therapy™ (TFT) and later learned the Tapas Acupressure Technique.

The author developed a clinically based theory of brain process and behavior to explain EMDR, and later extended the theory to all his treatment techniques. The theory or metaphor is accepted easily by patients, explains most of the phenomena observed in TFT, EMDR and other therapies, accounts for the formation of the entire personality and unusual phenomena, and is extremely useful in therapy.

Issues Work Sheet

List each Issue, develop the Aspects, if any, and write down the Phrases. Then number the Issues and Aspects as described in the book. Remember, assign 1 to the least Hurt.

Iss. No.	Issue	Asp. No.	Aspect	Phrase
——	——————	——	————————————	———————
——	——————	——	————————————	———————
——	——————	——	————————————	———————
——	——————	——	————————————	———————
——	——————	——	————————————	———————
——	——————	——	————————————	———————
——	——————	——	————————————	———————
——	——————	——	————————————	———————
——	——————	——	————————————	———————
——	——————	——	————————————	———————
——	——————	——	————————————	———————
——	——————	——	————————————	———————
——	——————	——	————————————	———————
——	——————	——	————————————	———————
——	——————	——	————————————	———————
——	——————	——	————————————	———————
——	——————	——	————————————	———————
——	——————	——	————————————	———————
——	——————	——	————————————	———————
——	——————	——	————————————	———————
——	——————	——	————————————	———————
——	——————	——	————————————	———————
——	——————	——	————————————	———————
——	——————	——	————————————	———————
——	——————	——	————————————	———————
——	——————	——	————————————	———————
——	——————	——	————————————	———————
——	——————	——	————————————	———————
——	——————	——	————————————	———————
——	——————	——	————————————	———————
——	——————	——	————————————	———————
——	——————	——	————————————	———————

To Purchase:

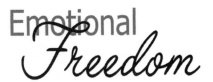
Emotional Freedom

Purchase this book from **Book Clearing House**:
- Telephone: 1800 431-1579 (24-hour service)
- Web site: http://www.bookch/psych.htm#9504
  (A secure credit card web site)

Due in 2004, a book teaching

The Process Healing Method
by Garry A. Flint, Ph.D.

This book describes a respectful treatment technique that easily heals all anxiety related mental health issues. It does this by organizing an internal treatment team. When all team members agree, the subconscious learns the tapping treatment. The book is full of treatment strategies for difficult issues.

For details and a free course about how to do it,
See: http://www.process-healing.com

For Research related to EFT and Process Healing,
See: http://www.process-healing.com/research.htm